KT-453-774

Contents

Work Based Learning in Primary Care

Edited by

Jonathan Burton

Associate Dean
Department of Postgraduate GP Education
London Deanery

and

Neil Jackson

Dean of Postgraduate GP Education
London Deanery

Radcliffe Medical Press

Radcliffe Medical Press Ltd
18 Marcham Road
Abingdon
Oxon OX14 1AA
United Kingdom

www.radcliffe-oxford.com
The Radcliffe Medical Press electronic catalogue and online ordering facility.
Direct sales to anywhere in the world.

British Library Cataloguing in Publication Data

A catalogue record for this book is available from the British Library.

ISBN 1 85775 996 6

Typeset by Aarontype Ltd, Easton, Bristol
Printed and bound by TJ International Ltd, Padstow, Cornwall

About the authors

The editors

Jonathan Burton
Associate Dean
Department of Postgraduate GP Education
London Deanery
General Practitioner

Neil Jackson
Dean of Postgraduate GP Education
London Deanery

The contributors

Hugh Barr
Professor Emeritus in Interprofessional Education
School of Integrated Health
University of Westminster

Reed Bowden
Associate Dean
Department of Postgraduate GP Education
London Deanery (until 2003)
General Practitioner

Yvonne Carter
Professor and Head of Department of General Practice and Primary Care
Barts and The London
Queen Mary's School of Medicine and Dentistry

Maggie Falshaw
Practice Manager
Limehouse Practice, London

Pamela Jackson
Community Nurse
Hertfordshire

Deirdre MacCarthy
Practice Nurse for 18 years
North Essex

Patrick MacCarthy
Former General Practitioner
North Essex

Penny Morris
Senior Lecturer in Communication Skills
School of Medicine, University of Leeds
Associate Dean
Department of Postgraduate Education
London Deanery

John Schofield
General Practitioner
North Essex
Associate Dean for Quality & Audit
Department of Postgraduate GP Education
London Deanery (until 2003)

Vicky Souster
Education Consultant
South London Organisation of Vocational Training Schemes (SLOVTS)
Former Practice Nurse

John Toby
General Practitioner
Chairman
Joint Committee on Postgraduate Training for General Practice

Penny Trafford
General Practitioner
Edgware, London
Associate Dean
Department of Postgraduate GP Education
London Deanery

Acknowledgements

Jonathan Burton and Neil Jackson

The ideas for this book stem from our many years of experience as GPs and educators. The list of educational colleagues who have helped us in our understanding of work based learning is long but in particular we would like to mention John Horder, Michael Carmi, Alex Jamieson, Vicky Souster, Steve Hiew and Nalliah Sivananthan. We both owe a debt of gratitude to our colleagues at the Limes Medical Centre in Epping and the Elizabeth Courtauld Surgery in Halstead, who have taught us so much about work based learning.

The chapter authors in this book have all been prepared to review and edit their writing, which has meant extra work for them, but we hope that the collective result is seen as more cohesive. We extend our thanks to them for their commitment and patience.

We would like to acknowledge the untiring support of Pam Roue, Debbie Torrie and Sue Hogarth at the London Deanery. We thank them for their help. Gillian Nineham has been a fantastically encouraging editor and has been generous in the giving of her time to this project.

Lastly we would like to thank those who have read and commented on our text: these include John Launer and Gillian Nineham. In particular we would like to thank our wives, Kathryn Burton and Pamela Jackson, for the support they have offered us during this project.

Glossary

Appraisal	Usually periodic performance review, but as applied to GPs is being seen as facilitated professional development within set parameters
Bandolier	Free but serious journal on evidence based clinical practice
BNF	*British National Formulary* – authoritative handbook on prescribed drugs, published six-monthly
CAIPE	UK Centre for the Advancement of Interprofessional Education – a non-governmental think-tank
CHD	Coronary heart disease
Cochrane Library	Authoritative library of healthcare research
CPD	Continuing professional development
CPP	Committee on Professional Performance (within GMC)
CQI	Continuous quality improvement
Dean or Director of GP Education	Medically qualified manager of GP education in a geographical area
Deanery	Department for GP education
DENs	Doctors' educational needs
DfID	Department for International Development – UK government department
DH or DoH	Department of Health (government department)
ECDL	European Computer Driving Licence
EMQ	Extended matching question
GMC	General Medical Council
GMS	General Medical Services – one type of contract for practices
HA	Health authority
HbA1c/fructosamine	Measures of diabetic control
HEA	Health Education Authority
IM&T	Information management and technology
LMC	Local medical committee – local branches of the BMA
LOTs	Local organising teams – related to work of the HEA
MCQ	Multiple choice question
Medline/Pubmed	Databases of journal articles

Mentor	Computerised textbook
MEQ	Modified essay question
MIQUEST	Instrument for searching and integrating electronic health data from one or more practice systems
MPET	Multiprofessional education and training
NCAA	National Clinical Assessment Authority – government body with responsibility for assessing doctors in trouble
NHSU	NHS University
OSCE	Objective structured clinical examination
PACT	NHS system for collecting and analysing prescribing data
PCG	Primary care group – management unit for primary care in a geographical area: now phased out
PCT	Primary care trust – management unit for primary care in a geographical area
PDP	Personal development plan – record of personal learning for a GP
PHCT	Primary healthcare team
PMS	Personal Medical Services – one type of contract for practices
Portfolio	Record of personal learning (mandatory for nurses)
PPDP	Practice professional development plan – learning plan for a practice
PUNs	Patients' unmet needs
RCGP	Royal College of General Practitioners
SP	Simulated patient
WBL	Work based learning
WDC	Workforce Development Confederation

Introduction

Jonathan Burton and Neil Jackson

Our interest

We have had a long interest in work based learning (WBL). Our interest started when we were young GPs and became involved, separately and unknown to each other, in practice based learning. For most of our careers, we have combined clinical practice with educational work, and it is through the latter that we first met one another. The idea for this book came from our long interest and involvement in practice based learning and other forms of WBL. In trying to describe and understand WBL, we really want to describe two different processes: what and how people learn and how they turn or should turn that learning into improving their performance at work.

External and internal influences on WBL

Learning is not divorced from the external realities of life, such as government policy and directives: indeed these realities drive the agenda of change and greatly influence what is learned, by whom and for what purpose. Many external influences will have a bearing on the quality of WBL. These are the influences of the audit society, and for that reason the book does address issues of quality (evidence based practice in Chapter 10, clinical governance in Chapter 9) at some length.

There are internal realities too. Potential opportunities for learning occur daily at work. Individuals may keep their knowledge up to date by a number of expedient learning methods, which they may hardly recognise as learning, reading around subjects and discussing cases with colleagues on a need-to-know basis. Motivation and organisation are everything here and individuals may feel too hard-pressed to pursue all these options. Much may be left unlearned. Teamwork, involving work colleagues, influences how and what individuals learn for themselves: team members may teach each other explicitly and, as

Chapter 6 shows, such activity will occur across professional boundaries. Much of the book focuses on the way in which a culture conducive to learning can be created. The partial or total failure to create such a culture is also widely described, especially in Chapter 8. The immediate concerns of individual healthcare workers, and the teams in which they work, contribute great creative energy to the process of WBL and an account of the intrapersonal and interpersonal dynamic in work based learning forms a major part of the book.

Whose learning is described in this book?

This book does not have a primary purpose of proving that WBL in primary care is more effective than any other form of learning. WBL is not going to stop or start because it is worse or better than other forms of learning. It happens anyway – it is inescapable. What we hope to do with this book, therefore, is to describe what it is, how it works and what makes it successful. In order to uncover, describe and communicate as many of these different processes as we can, we have made wide use of personal accounts of learning and for much of the book these accounts cover the experiences of all members of the primary care team.

Many of these are in the published literature, and are referenced. Others (often fictionalised) come from authors' experiences, either in their teaching work or in their clinical work. Such examples are normally not referenced. Wherever quotations or accounts are in italics, then the italicised section represents the actual words of learners or the actual text from cited publications.

One profession that has experienced a great role change over the last 15 years has been nursing. Many nurses have learned entirely new skills, skills which are appropriate for their roles in the management of chronic diseases, and so on. Such a sea change is part of the story of WBL. However, learning is not just a matter of changing one's own capacity or improving one's own performance. The delivery of care depends on the whole team – how they work together and who does what. Clinical and non-clinical staff are all part of the team.

Although this book is about primary care, some of the chapters (particularly Chapter 5 on apprenticeship and Chapter 8 on poor performance) describe the world of doctors only. The reader can, hopefully, extrapolate some general principles from these chapters. Much of what is written on apprenticeship in Chapter 5 could be applied to the forms of practice based attachments that are now being rolled out as part of the training for nurse practitioners and healthcare assistants. Equally, some of the educational concomitants of poor performance in doctors – for example, failure to keep up to date in knowledge, and ineffective involvement in peer- and self-assessment – could be applied to poor performance in nurses and other professional groups.

The promise of information technology

The role of information technology (IT) in work based learning is constantly underlined and is mentioned in all the chapters in this book except Chapter 11.

For hundreds of years, since the invention of the printing press, verbal literacy has underpinned the spread of factual knowledge and ideas throughout society. We are now in a period of transition. Computer literacy begins to offer us an alternative to verbal literacy, an alternative that promises to be more effective. Computers open up a whole world of factual knowledge and ideas, but they also offer a way of recording and quantifying WBL performance and can give easily accessed feedback. Technology has become an integral part of everyday life in pre-registration teaching, hospitals and general practice.

IT skills for healthcare professionals have become increasingly important in the new NHS: for example, IT skills can be used in literature searching, evidence based medicine, problem solving, etc. In addition, self-directed learning, critical thinking, and integration of theory and practice can be enhanced through IT. There is a need to ensure through the work based learning process that healthcare professionals use electronic tools appropriately and effectively in contributing to their continuing professional development as individuals and team members. This also applies on a larger scale to team learning and organisational development.

The future

At the end of the book, we look at where WBL in primary care should go next. We consider how WBL could be made more effective, and, in particular, consider the role of the objective review of performance (known broadly as assessment) in promoting change and improvement. At the same time, we are mindful of the essentially creative nature of WBL within primary care teams and the danger of imposing too many straitjackets upon it.

With the advent of a large and significant government programme of primary care development and the formation of primary care trusts (PCTs) we also wish to emphasise the relevance of WBL in developing the future strategy for education and training in primary care. WBL can also facilitate learning across professional and organisational boundaries, i.e. across the primary and secondary care sectors in the NHS.

CHAPTER 1

Theory and practice of work based learning and why work based learning in the new NHS

Jonathan Burton and Neil Jackson

Work is the curriculum. (Boud[1])

Introduction

Most of the writing about WBL comes from departments of higher education and has as its particular aim the need to examine the relationship between WBL and certificated learning within higher education.[1,2] WBL in primary care is largely an informal activity, undertaken by almost all healthcare workers. Much of the time it has little connection with academic qualifications. However, properly structured and certificated learning should be seen as a key part of WBL when professionals need to acquire a completely new set of skills.

We believe that, important as it is at the moment, WBL will become increasingly important in the next few years as the focus on performance and quality in the workplace grows.

Learning is influenced by what is happening at work. The influences are not just the random encounters with patients, but also the way in which the practice attempts to adjust itself to what are ever-changing expectations in healthcare. New forms of accessing knowledge (such as computer based learning) will transform the potential of WBL, while older approaches will be improved and made more sophisticated. And, as later chapters will show, WBL is not only based on the collaborative activity of learning together. It has the potential to contribute *to* collaborative and supportive relationships at work.

Relatively little has been written about WBL in primary care and access to the original research on which the general literature is based is not easily accessible to those working in primary care. The purpose of this chapter, therefore, is to set out briefly for the reader some of theory about work based learning, and to describe the various approaches to work based learning which are used, on a daily basis, in primary care.

What is WBL?

WBL is central to lifelong learning. Most health professionals working in primary care are already formally or informally involved in work based learning.

Definitions of WBL come from the world of higher education. The definition that we have found most useful and have discussed before is that of Seagraves.[3,4] He describes WBL as linking learning to the work role through three different processes:

- learning *for* work
- learning *at* work
- learning *from* work.

This definition describes how learning takes place – what is called a process definition. Other definitions are related to the intention of WBL, relating WBL to performance,[5] or seeing it as a developmental necessity to help professionals build on the knowledge gained, historically, from their basic training.[6]

Most work based learning in primary care is experiential. There are two other aspects of work based learning, the deliberate approach and the dissemination approach.

WBL: the experiential approach

Most learning opportunities come from the actual day-to-day occurrences which are related to work. In general, these will occur at the place of work, but not always. Some will occur outside of work, but their potential influence is not diminished by that fact. A feature of experiential learning is that it creates a learning opportunity by causing uncertainty or puzzlement. This can be illustrated by this vignette from Hiew and Sivananthan.[7]

S, a practice nurse, encountered her uncle in a supermarket. He asked her opinion about a screening test for prostate cancer, PSA (prostate specific antigen), about which he had read in a magazine. S bluffed but felt uncomfortable, and realised that she could be asked the same again by patients attending her clinic. She consulted the GP she worked with, who was also embarrassed to have no answer. After openly discussing the problem in the group, they looked up the *Effective Healthcare* bulletin. They found the advice was provided in a professionals' version and a patients' version. The finding was taken back to the practice. At the long-term review of the learning group, S recalled that one year later an old man did come to ask about PSA. She gave him the patients' leaflet and the man decided for himself whether to have the test.

In this account S first realised she had a learning deficit *from* a work experience (although the encounter occurred in the supermarket, she was still in her professional role). She bluffed to cover up her lack of clear knowledge. S was lucky enough to be a member of a learning group, which met in her practice, and she was able to take her puzzling encounter to the learning group. This was learning *at* work. The discussion and further reading led to improved knowledge, which she was able to exercise for the benefit of a future patient. At a later meeting of the learning group there was a further discussion of this experience and the subsequent learning that came from it. All this subsequent learning was learning *for* work. Members of the group would probably have been encouraged by the useful outcome from this initially difficult experience and many would have renewed their own confidence in this area of practice.

There are other approaches to experiential learning which use the initial experience of uncertainty or puzzlement as the stimulus to learning. A formalised model for such an approach has been developed by Eve.[8] Richard Eve calls his system PUNs (patients' unmet needs) and DENs (doctors' educational needs) or PUNs and PENs (practitioners' educational needs). Learners using this system keep a written log in their office or consulting room. When the learner feels confused, puzzled, uncertain or dissatisfied with what has gone on, the learner records the event in his or her log. The initial learning opportunity can then be converted into useful learning, through personal study or in a group setting. Richard Eve recognises that deficits may exist in the following areas:

- clinical knowledge
- non-clinical knowledge
- skill
- attitude
- practice organisation.

Thomas describes in detail a work based approach to learning in which non-clinical as much as clinical problems form the core of the learning agenda.[9]

> *We have been able to undertake practice based learning on clinical or nonclinical matters. The team decides the learning agenda for each meeting, according to what is happening – or not happening – at the practice.*

So, in summary, experiential work based learning can occur as part of self-study or as part of group based study, can be based on a variety of clinical and non-clinical happenings and can involve learning *at, for* and *from* work.

WBL: the deliberate approach

Deliberate learning makes a very important contribution to WBL. There are limitations to what experiential learning can achieve if the knowledge base is insufficient. This is where deliberate learning comes in. The deliberate approach to work based learning assumes a planned approach to learning. It is this sort of learning which is more likely to be linked to academic qualifications. It is more likely to occur where the learner needs to acquire a new set of knowledge and skills for independent practice – such as in the case of a practice nurse undertaking training to cover sections of the practice workload independently. Here is a story of a practice nurse, illustrating this point.

> A practice nurse related how she had major responsibility for family planning in the practice. She had undertaken the family planning course some years previously, at a time when the practice had no female GP and when she had just started there as a practice nurse. She related how she was getting a lot of patients coming to her with female or gynaecology-related problems or for family planning advice, which she wasn't equipped for. Having been on the course she gradually developed the role of key practitioner in this area in the team.

Many people will find it difficult to see how going on a course can be seen as an example of WBL. Indeed, Hugh Barr addresses this very potential confusion, in Chapter 6, by defining such learning as work-related rather than work based.

Nevertheless, this family planning course was an example of learning *for* work. The knowledge and skills the nurse gained on the course have been used to increase her work based skills and her new capacities have become vital for the team's ability to serve its patients.

WBL: the dissemination approach

In a working team there is a pool of expertise. Some staff members will have areas of special competence and can be a source of information and explanation to their colleagues. Workers will go away on courses and updates and have new knowledge to share with their colleagues. Cases are often discussed at coffee or lunchtime. Someone may know the answer or, alternatively, everyone may realise, anew, that they are confused in a certain area, so one person's uncertainty has made them all aware of their own learning needs.

> One practice in the Practice Tutor scheme in Camden and Islington set time aside at its regular interprofessional practice learning sessions to hear from the participants about the courses they had attended since the last meeting. A GP commented on how useful this had been and how much the doctors had learned from the nurses' accounts of their training courses.

There is more about this scheme in the next chapter.

Informal discussions can be helpful. A nurse practitioner reported how she met with colleagues for such discussions after sessions in the practice.

> The discussions are informal and are possible because all the staff finish at the same time. All sorts of things are discussed – who to refer to, diagnostic problems, prescribing issues and so forth.

Dissemination of knowledge and experience from within the working team is widespread. It is usually unstructured. It is a hugely useful part of WBL but not everyone has the opportunity to benefit from it, especially those who work in small practices (and do not attend multipractice learning groups). In addition, as with all informal learning, there is a danger. Because such learning is informal and depends on what colleagues know, it may lead to the dissemination of unhelpful or even wrong information.

Dissemination of learning also occurs in a more formal setting: for example, when a colleague who may well be a member of the extended primary care team helps to show, on the basis of his or her own skills and knowledge, how a service to patients can be improved. An example of this would be the podiatrist showing the doctors and nurses in the primary care team how to examine the diabetic foot.

WBL: responding to complexity

The work environment seems to be becoming increasingly complex. Greater levels of knowledge and more skills are expected of health professionals, who, at the same time, may live in fear of failing in a seemingly impossible task. Patients know and expect more and no longer automatically defer to professionals. The health service is able to provide more services, and professionals need to know how to access these on behalf of their patients. This means knowing what other members of the immediate team can offer, and what other services are available further away. What one patient might want or need at any one time and what evidence based medicine prescribes for him or her – these may be at variance. The task for professionals is increasingly difficult in this complex world.

How can WBL contribute to the resolution of this complexity? First, it can help individuals cope with that succession of moments of puzzlement, uncertainty and ignorance. It can offer occasions for resolving puzzlement. WBL can make practice safer. Chapters 3 and 7 cover how this might happen in greater detail.

Our view is that WBL will increasingly be the major route by which lifelong learning will occur. It will be become more robust as practice learning and personal learning become more carefully thought through. Immediate access to appropriate knowledge, via the Internet and other resources, will help to make WBL more evidence based and less haphazard. The complexity of the working task will not diminish, but WBL will give a range of answers to resolving that complexity.

Why work based learning in the new NHS?

The emphasis on delivering quality standards in the new NHS has been frequently highlighted by the government in its various policy documents, e.g. *A First Class Service – quality in the new NHS*.[10] Key to the quality agenda is lifelong learning for all healthcare professionals to meet the challenge of a fast-changing world, medical advances, new technologies and new approach to patient care.

In the pursuit of lifelong learning in the NHS, models of education and training are required to give NHS staff a clear understanding of how their own roles integrate with those of others in the healthcare system.

In the government publication *Working Together, Learning Together – a framework for lifelong learning in the NHS*, the vision of patient-centred care in the NHS is dependent upon learning and development for all NHS healthcare professionals.[11] By a process of WBL the vision can be realised and healthcare professionals, teams and organisations can be enabled to acquire, sustain and develop appropriate knowledge, skills and attitudes to ensure quality patient care.

The NHS also invests a huge amount of public money each year (over £2.5 billion) in education and training for staff. Given this situation it is vital to ensure value for money and effective outcomes and the process of work based learning can greatly contribute to this.

The government has also declared its commitment to establishing the NHS University (NHSU) as from 2003, to enhance lifelong learning for NHS staff and, here again, WBL could have a significant part to play. A system of WBL for NHS staff would facilitate individual healthcare professionals in becoming more reflective and analytical in their approach to patient care. This in turn would enhance quality service provision. The process of lifelong learning can also be recognised and accredited within an academic framework. These and other additional benefits of WBL in the new NHS are summarised in Box 1.1.

Box 1.1: The benefits of WBL in the new NHS

- WBL enables a collaborative approach between institutes of higher education, employers and employees to the ultimate benefit of patients using the NHS.
- WBL promotes formal and informal collaborative learning at practice level.
- Learning which takes place at work can be given academic recognition while taking into account both present and future roles of employees.
- WBL can promote both individual and team development within NHS organisations.
- WBL should enable a balance to be achieved between personal fulfilment for individual healthcare professionals and the wider needs of the employing organisation and the NHS as a whole.
- WBL allows a flexible approach to the timing, location and methods of learning.
- WBL promotes self-motivation, critical thinking and reflective practice.
- WBL enhances a greater understanding of working within the complex environment of the new NHS.

References

1 Boud D and Solomon N (2001) *Work-based Learning. A new higher education.* Open University Press, Buckingham.

2 Brennan J and Little B (1996) *A Review of Work Based Learning in Higher Education.* Department for Education and Employment, Sheffield.

3 Seagraves L, Osborne N, Neal P *et al.* (1996) *Learning in Smaller Companies, final report.* University of Stirling, Stirling.

4 Burton J, Jackson N and McEwen Y (1999) GP tutors, work-based learning and primary care groups. *Education for General Practice.* **10**: 417–22.

5 Foster E (1996) *Comparable but Different: work-based learning for a learning society.* DfEE and University of Leeds, Leeds.

6 Eraut M (1994) *Developing Professional Knowledge and Competence.* Falmer Press, London.

7   Hiew S and Sivananthan N (2001) The partnership in progress in practice project. *J Learning Workplace*. **3**: 6–10. (www.tlw.org.uk)

8   Eve R (2002) Discovering learning needs with PUNs and DENs. *J Learning Workplace*. **4**: 9–11. (www.tlw.org.uk)

9   Thomas M (2001) PPDP meetings: a tool for learning. *Update*. 20 December. (www.tlw.org.uk)

10   Secretary of State for Health (1998) *A First Class Service – quality in the new NHS*. HMSO, London.

11   Secretary of State for Health (2001) *Working Together, Learning Together – a framework for lifelong learning in the NHS*. HMSO, London.

CHAPTER 2

The practice as a learning organisation

Neil Jackson and Jonathan Burton

The team that became great didn't start off great – it learned how to produce extra-ordinary results. (Senge[1])

Introduction

Over 90% of contacts between the population and the NHS take place in the primary care setting. This has resulted in increasing emphasis on a primary care-led NHS by successive governments over the past few years.[1,2] Such an emphasis has highlighted the need for a multiprofessional/multidisciplinary system of working in primary care. The principle of service provision and development in partnership with education and training has also been established. It should naturally follow that multidisciplinary learning will benefit multidisciplinary working. The general practice of the future will need to become a learning organisation to encourage healthcare professionals to work and learn together and develop as a team. To promote higher standards of patient care in the complexity of the new NHS such a team must be capable of adapting to change while sustaining its own development within the learning organisation.

Understanding how we can learn together, as a collective primary care team, is still a relatively new concept to many healthcare professionals.[3] It is important to recognise that it can only happen as a result of learning at the whole team level, rather than by training individual team members in isolation.

In addition, teams will succeed only if they address the quality agenda, and successful learning organisations will need to be aware of their responsibilities in all the components of clinical governance, which are summarised in Box 2.1.

Box 2.1: Components of clinical governance[4]

- Audit.
- Evidence based medicine.
- Significant event analysis.
- Risk management.
- Patient involvement.

The practice as a learning organisation

Learning organisations are possible because, deep down, we are all learners. No one has to teach an infant to learn. In fact, no one has to teach infants anything. They are intrinsically inquisitive, masterful learners who learn to walk, speak and pretty much run their households all on their own. Learning organisations are possible because not only is it our nature but we love to learn. Most of us at one time or another have been part of a great team, a group of people who functioned together in an extraordinary way – who trusted one another, who complimented each other's strengths and compensated for each other's limitations, who had common goals that were larger than individual goals, and who produced extraordinary results.

What they experienced was a learning organisation. The team that became great didn't start off great – it learned how to produce extraordinary results. (Senge[1])

Senge describes learning as a natural and enjoyable adventure, but team learning and team creativity do not arise spontaneously. They arise in response to systematic endeavour by teams to improve their work. We call the practice which has successfully adopted the ethos of the learning organisation a working-learning team. We are now going to describe the things that help to establish a working-learning team.

The characteristics of the working-learning team are many but they are certainly not hard to attain. It should be possible for any practice to be successful in this way. For example, in 1998, a group of some 20 GPs, most of whom came from non-teaching practices, identified a number of aspects of their own practices which contributed to their success as learning organisations (*see* Box 2.2).[4]

Box 2.2: Characteristics of the practice as a learning organisation[4]

1 Communication.
2 Peer support.

---

3 Peer learning.
4 Shared values.
5 An appropriate mixture of learning opportunities.
6 Some learning driven by practice team members' needs and occurring within the practice.
7 Some learning taking place outside the workplace and being disseminated through the practice.
8 Organisational factors, such as practice libraries and protected time for learning.

There are some practices that, in addition to serving the public, involve themselves in teaching and training young GPs, nurses and healthcare assistants, or they may be involved in research activity. Such practices are likely to thrive as working-learning teams. They expose themselves to outside stimuli through membership of educational or research networks. They have to submit themselves to external scrutiny in order to maintain their acceptability as teaching or research practices. In 1998, Carter, Jackson and Barnfield highlighted 12 characteristics of such learning practices which are reproduced in Box 2.3.[5]

Box 2.2 summarises the basic characteristics, the foundations without which practices cannot start their evolution from a group of disparate individuals working in the same place to a working-learning team. Box 2.3 summarises the characteristics of practices which go further and deliberately and strategically set out to create the best environment for working-learning.

Box 2.3: The 12 characteristics of the learning practice identified by Carter, Jackson and Barnfield[5]

- a training practice with an established ethos for medical, nursing and paramedical education and training which may be at an undergraduate or postgraduate level or both
- provides quality teaching in protected time
- demonstrates a firm partnership between service delivery and education
- utilises the process of education and training to manage the interface between service and research and development
- recognises the importance of primary care team development and the need for personal and professional development of each individual team member
- aspires to provide the highest possible standards of patient and population healthcare
- recognises the need for a multiprofessional/multidisciplinary approach to education and training

- subscribes to the concept that medical/non-medical education is a continuum
- fosters a culture of lifelong learning and reflective practice within a multiprofessional team
- uses evaluation/evidence as the basis for work
- is committed to forward thinking and innovation
- recognises the need to take some risks and accept some mistakes.

WBL and the successful working-learning team

As set out in Chapter 1, the definition of WBL in primary care is as follows. WBL occurs at work, from work and for work. In the next part of this chapter we will discuss practice and multipractice learning. We will look particularly at how collaborative learning can contribute to both individual and team outcomes and we will show how all three of the aspects of work based learning contribute to a more successful working-learning practice.

What makes the practice a successful learning organisation?

Success has to start from somewhere. In most of the written accounts of thriving practice learning cultures, there is clearly a system of leadership. This might arise from within the practices as part of their own culture or occur as a result of outside influence, as in the Practice Tutor scheme described below. The external forces of change, such as changes in government policy for the NHS, clearly influence the direction in which all practice teams travel. Practices can be stimulated to adopt change by being encouraged to undertake a new way of doing things. Such encouragement is clearly a task for NHS management. For example, McKee and Watts[6] described two Norfolk practices which were invited to participate in a scheme to develop their own practice professional development plans (PPDPs). These PPDPs were to be based on an assessment of learning needs. They were also to be attentive to the clinical governance agenda. The authors relate how at first the health service managers who were funding the study were doubtful that the practices could succeed, but the researchers concluded that:

> *Once the practices understood how to identify educational needs and their relation to clinical governance, they proved capable of proceeding autonomously in designing and exploring their own PPDPs.*[6]

Creative development of a practice team is also driven by the desire of its members to improve their services to patients: this is about the quality agenda. Many of the quality issues are summarised in Box 2.1, which details the components of clinical governance. In the end, everything is about quality – doing things well and being able to adjust and change good practice as circumstances change. Thomas describes the transformation of his practice by a team learning programme, which was based firmly on the clinical governance agenda.[7] He describes the sessions as being a discussion of '*what is happening – or not happening – at the practice*'. This is a story of how a practice was able to adopt and then own new ways of thinking about healthcare and then use these collectively to address issues of quality within the practice.

However, going back to Senge, it is through learning itself that the greatest change occurs. Modern trends in practice based learning have undoubtedly helped to build practices into working-learning teams. There is evidence that team learning can become a transforming experience, leading to improvements in working practices, communication and peer support. One of the biggest experiments in the UK in practice based learning has been the Practice Tutor scheme in Camden and Islington and Barnet. The Camden and Islington part of the scheme has been evaluated. It is this part that we will describe. Thirty practice learning groups were set up, representing roughly half the practices in Camden and Islington. Some groups were just made up of one practice. With smaller practices, groups were made up of more than one practice. Each group was led by a health professional from the participating practice(s). Peter Herbert has described the practice tutor scheme as a potentially addictive experience for the involved practices.[8]

The intention was to create a movement in self-directed learning which would become addictive, so that practices not used to meeting would become unable to function so well without their regular meetings under the scheme.

The evaluation of the scheme[9] showed that:

The evidence is that the Practice Tutor scheme successfully stimulates and manages the learning process. The evaluation identifies a range of benefits and outcomes of the Practice Tutor scheme. It provides an impetus to get going with practice based education, protected time for meeting, a forum for developing practice protocols and guidelines and for team building. It also provides a forum for training for specific skills, for sharing learning from other educational activities (conferences etc.) with colleagues, and, in some groups, peer support. The outcomes identified by participants are a change in practice culture so that education is an accepted part of it, more consistency of practice between team members, changes in referral and prescribing practice, development of new services and improved co-ordination of existing services.

The Practice Tutor scheme was set up with no precise rules, but participants were encouraged to follow an ethos based on voluntarism, self-directedness, interprofessionalism and the importance of protected time. The tutor's role was defined in simple terms and ideas for the tutor's support were set out in a liberal and non-prescriptive way.[7]

The evaluation showed that many of the aims were well achieved. In particular, 90% of the meetings were attended by staff from a variety of disciplines, and, at least in some of the teams, there was a very positive experience from the interprofessional learning. While the evaluators were cautious and chose not to claim that the scheme had led to dependable and measurable outcomes, their descriptions of what actually happened in participating practices suggested that things were achieved which just would not have happened if the scheme had not existed. Practices were able to harness problems in practice to learning opportunities. Common sense dictated that difficult and serious situations must be addressed. For example:

> *We have a planning meeting every six months. At that meeting we write down a list of items that need discussion. And then that changes very often at the last moment because something else comes up – we're very reactive – for example, one of our patients died driving and was an epileptic. That brought up issues around fitness to drive and someone had to be a witness at the coroner's court, so the next week we had a meeting about this. We're more reactive than we are (attentive) to our list (of learning needs) . . .*[9]

Many practices discovered that formal learning programmes were no more important than the process of the dissemination of learning.

> *Then the nurses have been included and we realised that they were going to a lot of very good meetings, so they could bring information back into the practice that could be circulated.*[9]

The evaluation of the Practice Tutor scheme included accounts of many examples of the benefits to the team from practice based learning.

Clearly, too, individuals benefit from being in a shared learning environment. Self-study and shared learning are capable of changing practice, but shared learning is likely to work more effectively, as *none of us is as smart as all of us.*[10] As Box 2.4 shows, in a working-learning practice, four kinds of learning are important.[11] An individual, studying by him/herself, is able to improve knowledge, skills, abilities and competencies and undertake personal development. Collaborative enquiry, where learning can take place between people rather than on an individual basis, is recognised as one of the key factors that can transform working practices into working-learning practices and is known to contribute powerfully to personal learning.

Box 2.4: Four types of learning (from Pedler and Aspinwall[11])

- Knowledge.
- Skills, abilities, competencies.
- Personal development.
- Collaborative enquiry (problem solving).

More about collaborative enquiry

Collaborative enquiry is now widely recognised as a perfect background for progress in learning. We think that it is important to break the business of collaborative learning into its two main constituent parts: collaborative learning as an aid to personal reflection, and collaborative learning as an aid to transforming a team's working practices.

The first constituent part can be illustrated by looking at the new arrangements for personal learning for psychiatrists. Collaborative learning has been established as the milieu for their professional development. Psychiatrists are now expected to meet in peer groups to pre-plan, discuss and report on their own individual professional development needs. The aim is that each individual has available, in the group, objective opinion and support. Against this background, they can test their plan and monitor their progress.

The peer group acts as the giver of objective opinion and the giver of support. Others, analysing practice and interpractice learning groups in the primary care setting, have also emphasised the educational importance of group members' knowledge, experience and opinion and the support that the peer group offers to its individual members.[12,13] The seeking of objective opinion (i.e. evidence based) can be part of the ethos of the group.[12]

Support can best be defined as that which occurs when a setting has been established in which individuals feel valued and safe. As will be discussed in Chapter 3, practice based learning certainly does not guarantee that such a supportive setting has been established.

The second constituent part of collaborative learning is as an aid to transforming a team's working practices. A description of this is provided in Souster,[14] Burton[15] and in Chapter 10 in this book. Here the process moves very quickly from a review of, for example, knowledge in a particular area, through a review of performance in practice (for example, via audit), to an informed discussion about how to do things better. With the increasing use of audit and similar methods of review in learning, this model will become more widespread.

These two constituent parts of collaborative learning are set out in Table 2.1. Appropriate facilities and resources for learning in the practice should be made

Table 2.1: Features of collaborative learning in primary care

Collaborative learning as an aid to personal learning	Collaborative learning as an aid to transforming a team's working practice
Members of group offer experience, knowledge and objective opinion to the learner.	The group seeks to inform itself about practice: this may mean getting outside, expert opinion.
Members of group offer support to the learner.	The group judges its performance in the area under study: for example, via audit. Armed with this information the group quickly decides what needs to be done to improve performance.
Evaluation: more difficult in respect of personal learning.	Evaluation: easier in judging a team's working practice, as audit cycles and other easily accessible measurement instruments may be used. Computerised data very important here.

available for all members of the primary healthcare team, including practice nurses, practice receptionists, practice managers, doctors and other healthcare professionals. Members of the practice team are encouraged to manage their own learning and career development but this should be linked to the wider needs of the team in its multidisciplinary approach to delivering quality service provision. Although learning starts from the job itself for each individual team member, the team as a whole must adapt to learning more rapidly and with increased flexibility in a world of growing complexity and change. More and more, such opportunities of time are being provided via practice or primary care organisation 'shutdowns'. In these, cover is often provided for emergencies, and paid for by primary care organisations, allowing the practice teams to benefit from protected time for learning.

Multiprofessional/multidisciplinary working and learning in the practice learning organisation

The process of continuing education and training in the learning practice must sustain the development and meet the needs of both primary care staff and service provision for patients. The training needs of the primary care team of professionals must be properly assessed in order to ensure the provision of appropriate training programmes. Any training or educational support provided for the healthcare professionals either within or outwith the practice learning organisation itself will require evaluation by both teachers and students. This is essential to ensure that the education and training provision is appropriate to meet professional learning needs. Evaluation is also essential from a quality assurance perspective, both in terms of the education and training provided and the practice learning organisation as a whole. Here a system of accreditation/reaccreditation of the practice is essential. A good example of a framework for this is the postgraduate training practice for GP training which is evaluated on a regular basis by a multidisciplinary team of healthcare professionals. Another example of this is the 'contract review' which takes place annually for practices in the PMS scheme. Related to this is the need to develop primary care based research and the appropriate training of primary health team members to equip them to take forward the research agenda. This will enhance an evidence based health service for patients and facilitate a 'three systems' approach whereby service provision is supported and informed by education and training and research and development.

A shared commitment to lifelong learning and reflective practice by all team members in their daily working lives should feature prominently in the working-learning practice. Establishing this principle in such an environment will ensure a highly trained and skilled practice workforce capable of delivering quality service provision to its population of patients.

Workforce planning and development in primary care

In the developing multiprofessional environment of a primary care-led NHS there is an ever-growing need for the future to invest in the establishment of practice learning organisations. On a larger scale other healthcare organisations such as primary care trusts (PCTs) and acute and community NHS trusts have now developed increased awareness of the need to develop multiprofessional learning environments. The way forward in terms of establishing the 'right' workforce or the 'appropriate' team for the job lies in taking account of both the numbers of healthcare professionals and a properly integrated skill-mix, i.e. a system of workforce planning is required, as well as healthcare professionals working and learning together.

In the modernised NHS new structures and processes for an integrated multi-professional/multidisciplinary approach to healthcare delivery are now in place. Workforce Development Confederations (WDCs) have been established in England with the broad remit and responsibility for the workforce planning of all staff working in all sectors of healthcare, including primary care. In addition, their role will encompass human resource management issues, including recruitment and retention initiatives, and the quality assurance of non-medical education and training. As from April 2002 WDCs will manage the resources for education and training for all non-medical, undergraduate and postgraduate medical staff in the NHS through the MPET (Multiprofessional Education and Training) Levy. WDCs will also hold contracts with local education providers for pre-registration training for nurses, midwives and professionals allied to medicine. Following on from this is the need for practice placements for professional pre-registration and post-registration education in a variety of settings including primary care. Here once again the principles of the learning organisation should be applied to ensure both supervision and support for each trainee healthcare professional.

Within each WDC sector, PCTs have been established with funding to ensure the planning and commissioning of quality, seamless service provision for patients across the primary and secondary care sectors in their localities. These primary care organisations must also take responsibility for the strategic management of education and training of practices and their primary care staff within their boundaries.

Teaching PCTs are also being established in areas of social and health deprivation to provide an academic focus to support local recruitment and retention initiatives for general practitioners and other primary care professionals. They will have a key part to play in the future development of primary care.

With the advent of these new structures in the NHS comes the need for each one to adopt the core principles of the learning organisation. These principles are paramount for both GP practices and larger-scale NHS organisations. For each healthcare organisation its success or failure in meeting the challenge offered by the new NHS lies in the capabilities, skills and motivation of its staff members.

References

1 Senge PM (1992) *The Fifth Discipline – the art and practice of the learning organisation.* Century Business, London.

2 Secretary of State for Health (1996) *Primary Care: delivering the future.* HMSO, London.

3 Secretary of State for Health (1997) *The New NHS.* HMSO, London.

4 Burton J, Jackson N and McEwen Y (1999) GP Tutors, work-based learning and primary care groups. *Ed Gen Pract.* **10**: 417–22.

5 Carter Y, Jackson N and Barnfield A (1998) The learning practice: a new model for primary health care teams. *Ed Gen Pract.* **9**: 182–8.

6 McKee A and Watts M (2002) Practice and professional development plans: a project from Norfolk. *J Learning Workplace.* **4**: 6. (www.tlw.org.uk and www.uea.ac.uk/care/research/PPDP)

7   Thomas M (2002) PPDP: a tool for learning. First published in *Update*, 20 December 2001. Available in full in the 2002 volume of *J Learning Workplace*. (www.tlw.org.uk)

8   Herbert P (2002) The Practice Tutor Scheme in Camden and Islington and South Barnet. *J Learning Workplace*. **4**: 7–9. www.tlw.org.uk (accessed 16 June 2002).

9   Russell J, Rogers S and Modell M (2002) Evaluation report on the Camden and Islington Practice Tutor Scheme. *J Learning Workplace*. (www.tlw.org.uk)

10 Bennis W and Biederman P (1997) *Organizing Genius: the secrets of creative collaboration.* Addison-Wesley, Reading, MA.

11 Pedler M and Aspinwall K (1995) *'Perfect plc?' The purpose and practice of organizational learning.* McGraw-Hill, London.

12 Hiew S and Sivananthan N (2001) The partnership in progress in practice project. *J Learning Workplace*. **3**: 6–10. (www.tlw.org.uk)

13 Burton J (1998) Multipractice, self-directed learning groups in North Thames East Region. *Ed Gen Pract*. **9**: 512–16.

14 Souster V (1999) Tailor made practice. *J Learning Workplace*. **1**: 2–7. (www.tlw.org.uk)

15 Burton J (1997) Locality learning. *CAIPE Bulletin*. **13**: 27–8.

CHAPTER 3

Work based learning in action: collaborative learning and personal learning

Jonathan Burton

She is made good by getting an intelligent insight into her own work.
(Xenophon, c 435–c 354 BC)

Introduction

In this chapter I have set out to describe the ways in which nurses, doctors and practice managers tackle the task of learning.

The writing in this chapter is based on interviews, stories and practical accounts from others and from my own experience in practice.

In the early part of the chapter I describe the public and private agendas for learning and the interrelationship between collaborative learning and personal learning. I then go on to discuss collaborative learning and personal learning in detail, including a look at some of their problems. Finally I make some suggestions as to how such learning could be made more efficient. This chapter is not a paean of praise to those who are improving their services to patients. It is an attempt to try and describe what works for learners.

As this chapter describes nurses, doctors and managers, I have tried to be even handed and not to assume that the efforts or work of any one group is more important. Nor have I dealt with the special arrangements for promoting or monitoring educational progress in any one of these professions, which are beyond the scope of this chapter.

All the accounts on which this chapter is based are reports from professionals of how they have set about their learning. Some of these accounts are celebrations of achievement, but sometimes there are descriptions of difficulties. At the end I will reflect on what is working at present and suggest how lifelong learning can be made more effective, while remaining sustainable.

A changing world: challenge and problem

The world in which health professionals are learning has changed immensely in the last two decades. Nurses in particular are taking on roles of major responsibility for patient care, and expectations of quality are increasing year by year. For some, this changing culture is full of promise and challenge,[1] and in meeting the challenge many teams have enjoyed a sense of achievement. The experience is not, however, totally fulfilling and the discordance between personal interests/concerns and external forces/events has to become part of the story of learning. In undertaking WBL, individuals and teams do have to face both ways: towards the external reality of the world and to the inner reality of personal concerns and responses. Successful WBL should mean two things: first, that individuals and teams achieve success in mastering the tasks of the moment and, second, that individuals (and the teams they make up) feel integrated, supported and understood.

The three motivations: personal, professional and service

When Sylvia Debreczeny undertook her study of primary care tutors and their relationship with the chief executives of primary care groups, she found that philosophical differences between managers and professional educators were common.[2] On many occasions, each side was in an entrenched position – unable to understand the other's point of view. She saw that she could clarify this situation by describing learning as being driven by any one (or sometimes a combination) of three motivations. The first motivation was personal – what interested the learner. The second was professional – learning that took place in accordance with the standards and recommendations of a professional group (such as the Royal College of Nursing). And the third was service-led – often associated with the modernisation of the NHS. For example, it might be to do with the management of information, or with nationally prescribed ways of managing chronic diseases, or with local issues, or with the quality agenda, or with evidence based healthcare, and so on. In some situations the personal, the professional and the service-led orientations might share common ground or even identical ground. Individual learners could learn for personal satisfaction *and* learn in order to satisfy service requirements.

At times, individuals might value their personal interests more than those that are dictated by the service. For many individuals personal and service interests are identical, whilst for others they are not.[1] Such interests keep some practitioners sane, enthused and refreshed. Many examples of this are given by Linden West, who describes how practitioners' individual clinical interests – like studying herbalism – help sustain morale in difficult circumstances.[3] But it would be a mistake to define the personal and the service-led as incompatible – far from it. The following story is condensed from an article in *Medeconomics*. It illustrates how an erstwhile 'Cinderella' area of practice has become one of current importance, and how what was initially a personal interest has now become a mainstream one.[4]

> Dr F started seeing addicts in her first week in practice, and looking back says it was not a conscious decision. She had no specialist training but wanted to help them and learned on the job. That was many years ago, and now she is a national figure in this area. She has come to understand that most users are better managed in primary care and sees addiction as a chronic illness like any other chronic illness. She now trains other GPs and health workers locally and nationally, acts as a supervising mentor on the College of GPs course, and sits on national bodies. This area of practice is now regarded as one in which GPs should become specialists within the new NHS.

The boundaries between personal, professional and service-led are often indistinct and what starts as a personal interest or activity may become accepted as a contribution to the professional and service-led agenda in time. As always, a long-term view of such matters is the right view.

Features of work based learning in action

Definition and description of collaborative learning

Learning is undertaken in a social context, involving interaction with others. Such 'learning together' activity is often called collaborative learning. This term covers one-on-one and group learning experiences: collaborative learning can be formal and informal. Collaborative learning is integral to WBL, as so much of work is delivered by teams.

Definition and description of personal learning

Personal learning can be defined as that learning which is undertaken by individuals in response to their own learning needs. Personal learning is often a solitary activity. There are reasons for this. It is practical to learn by oneself, fitting in the learning to the nooks and crannies of a busy working day. But, more importantly, personal learning is driven by work based experiences, experiences which are unique to the individual. Frequently, in the course of a working day, the health professional sees a patient and thinks: I need to read up on that or discuss that with so and so. Opportunities for learning arise from such unique experiences.

The links between personal and collaborative learning

Personal and collaborative learning are inextricably linked. Collaborative learning contributes towards the increase in personal knowledge and skills, and the influence of others is almost a necessity if we are to learn to change our own attitudes. Conversely, what has been learned through personal study or reflection is the foundation of each individual's contribution to collaborative learning. Personal learning can be validated and enriched and personal beliefs challenged if the learner has the opportunity to benefit from the opinions and experiences of peers. Others can lend support, give objective opinions, speak from their own experience.

Many health professionals like to share their work and learning experiences with colleagues. They feel that this form of shared learning is practical and, in a trusting relationship, helpful.

It is also a practical necessity to integrate personal learning with team learning. Teams need to build relationships, to understand each other's work and to discuss ways of improving the joint delivery of care to groups of patients. A formal direction towards the integration of individual learning for GPs and team learning has been given by the Chief Medical Officer's report of 1998.[5] This report proposed a more purposeful way of undertaking personal learning and acknowledged that personal learning should be integrated into the development of the practice as a whole. A good example of how this integration has taken place is reported by Staley.[6]

Practices and the individuals in them are influenced by what others are doing. Sharing and comparing achievements with others is a stimulus to change. We all need to give ourselves the opportunity to see when we have got behind. Such opportunities may arise from being appropriately self-critical, from comparing one's practices with those of a work colleague or by undertaking a more rigorous approach to peer review, ideally involving an arbiter of good practice.

A nurse practitioner was asked about how her practice team had been influenced by doing comparative audits with neighbouring practices. The audits had been set up by five practices in one geographical locality (which in turn had been advised by a consultant in public health). She was able to describe how, from these comparative audits, her practice team had found that they had measured most of the 'at risk' cardiac disease patients' lipids but they hadn't done much about it – in terms of considering drug treatment. This had 'stuck out' and had engendered a determination to change things – and that was being done at the moment.

Many practices and individuals, however, are not exposed to this type of peer influence. They then run the risk of becoming adrift and in more serious cases of being identified as poorly performing. This type of situation is analysed in greater detail in Chapter 8.

Difficulty of separating collaborative learning from personal learning

It is difficult to separate personal learning from collaborative learning. The aspiration for personal development is often tied up with what happens in the team, and colleagues continually exercise an influence on how we think and how we estimate our own proficiency in the various aspects of our working roles. It is difficult to separate the interpersonal (what goes on between people) from the intrapersonal (what goes on within a person). Whenever this chapter addresses the intrapersonal aspects of learning, the reader will be aware, through the various arguments and accounts, that the influences of others on personal learning are strong and pervasive.

Characteristics of collaborative learning

The characteristics of collaborative learning are summarised in Box 3.1.

Box 3.1: Characteristics of collaborative learning

1 Can be formal or informal.
2 Can involve two or more people.
3 The same individuals can be in turn benefactors and beneficiaries of collaborative learning.
4 Has its own discordancies.

Informal collaborative learning

Quite often colleagues in a working team will consult each other, at coffee, in the corridor or by seeking out emergency help – perhaps a knock on the door and a request for help on a puzzling situation. These are the informal approaches. Such approaches may be based on one person's view of the other's expertise, or may simply be a wish to sort out uncertainties in the spirit of joint enquiry. John Launer and I, in writing about clinical supervision, have described these common but largely undocumented approaches as 'native' to primary care.[7] They are widely and routinely used, and are vital in the overall pattern of learning. Most readers who work in primary care will recognise how much they themselves depend on such experiences for their own learning. They are practical, easy to employ and in most cases a contribution to better patient care. Informal one-on-one collaborative learning may be based on one party's knowledge that the other party has some particular expertise.

An example of such an encounter involved a corridor meeting between a GP and a practice nurse.

> The GP had never undertaken spirometry on patients, a task that the practice nurse routinely did and had been trained to do. He had been asked about the process by another professional and realised his ignorance so he kept his puzzlement in the back of his mind. He met the practice nurse in the corridor of the practice and he was able to discuss spirometry with her for a couple of minutes and his specific questions were answered.

Equally, one-on-one collaborative learning may start off by being a question from one party to another, but may act as a learning spur to both. Here are some examples of such an interaction.

> A practice nurse asked a GP why some patient groups were to be immunised with Pneumovax. What was pneumococcus and why were some patients vulnerable? He felt unable to answer her questions fully and went away to read up the subject. He also photocopied a review article from *Update* which he gave to her.

> A practice nurse was undertaking a cervical smear on a patient. The patient had an area of chronic infection in the groin, and the nurse asked the GP to look at it. The GP recognised the syndrome but she could not remember its name. At coffee time the two of them looked through some dermatology books and recognised the syndrome as hidradenitis suppurativa. The nurse had never heard of it and the GP knew about it, had seen it several times in the past, but was still somewhat vague about it. For example, she had not remembered its name, nor could she say precisely what sort of treatments were recommended.

These brief vignettes illustrate the potency of informal collaborative learning. It is the fact that such learning episodes take place within the framework of ordinary working life, and use the interplay between working colleagues, that makes them so important. Resolution of puzzlement often requires little time and no great effort. Collaborative learning of this sort is probably one of the main ways in which significant work based learning occurs. The writing by educationalists on collaborative learning has emphasised the way in which collaborative learning adds benefit.[8] Two people learning together achieve more learning than two separate individuals working apart – as Bennis and Biederman say, *'none of us is as smart as all of us'*.[9]

Formal collaborative learning

More and more practice teams are involved in formal practice educational meetings, and such meetings are increasingly undertaken in protected time. For example, the primary care organisation may pay for urgent calls to be covered during an afternoon learning session. Learning groups may also be run for the benefit of groups of professionals from more than one practice: such approaches are particularly appropriate for smaller practices.[10] Learning groups almost certainly need to be led, if they are to be effective. Leadership may be administrative, facilitatory or expert[11] – in the former situation, the leader arranges the meeting, but does not take a key role in helping the educational process. A facilitator, on the other hand, may help the learning process in a number of ways (*see* Box 3.2). Educational leadership may be from within the practice team – or it may come from outside and the facilitator may not have a clinical qualification.

Box 3.2: Educational leadership of WBL learning groups

1	Administrative	May only address the structural elements – for example, arranging the meeting, helping with papers and handouts.
2	Facilitatory	May address the learning process – taking responsibility for maintaining the involvement of the group members or keeping to established ground rules; helping the process of learning; may steer the learning group towards attention to outcome; is usually on an equal professional footing with the group members, but may have received some educational training.

3 Expert	Unusual in the primary care setting, but an example would be an individual who had been trained to lead a Balint group, and upon whose greater knowledge or skills the group would depend.

There are many ways of running learning groups. One of the most popular approaches is to have a programme of subjects to be covered, often with outside experts speaking. In a sense such an approach to learning is instructional rather than collaborative, but if the learning is work based, and orientated to improving work practices, then it is collaborative, because the learners have joint responsibility for turning new knowledge, skills and attitudes into improvements in practice. Learning groups may also address work based issues but without outside experts helping. Frequently such meetings are case based[10] or situation based.[12] Case based and situation based meetings very often allow discussion of difficult situations which have arisen in practice and are therefore orientated to the clinical governance agenda. This has already been discussed in Chapter 2.

The advantages for learners of being in a learning group are many. There is evidence that learning groups are good for morale.[13] One outcome of collaborative learning is that learners can aspire to adopt what they see as the better practices demonstrated by their peers.[10,11] Learners can return on a cyclical basis to core themes and can use audit figures to indicate whether they are jointly improving their care of patients, and, where they are not, can decide together what should be done to remedy the situation. Such learning sessions are in fact learning-and-action sessions, because the discussion and learning lead to decisions about better forms of practice, all within the same block of one to two hours. The area of cyclical and comparative audit as a tool for improved performance is covered in Chapter 10. Finally, there are some really practical issues. Performance outcomes are increasingly likely to be contractual for primary care teams and it will be almost impossible for a practice to manage outcome-related contracts without having learning-and-action sessions. In-practice learning groups have therefore been given life and purpose by the way primary healthcare is being developed.

Discordancies of collaborative learning

However, there are potential discordancies in collaborative learning. In learning groups, there may be too few or no ground rules. The meeting may therefore be unproductive or, worse, some learners may feel abused. To make the meetings productive there should be a clear and agreed structure, and there should be an attention to outcomes. All group members should be able to answer these two questions: what is the point of these meetings and what do I/ we want to get out of them? If the answers to such questions are uncertain, then there may be little point in having any meetings unless the format is improved. To prevent meetings being abusive, approaches to personal safety should be established. After all, in such groups, matters of personal performance and competence may be discussed either implicitly or explicitly. These are areas of great and often secret personal concern. A learning group probably loses more by leaving one or two of its members bruised than it gains by temporary advances in 'productivity'. As learning groups and working teams are often made up of the same people, it does not pay to leave individuals feeling bad as a result of an imperfect learning experience, or one which has made them feel persecuted or belittled.

> One GP reported how she felt inadequate during the learning sessions in her practice. She felt so far behind her 'brilliant partners' that her experience was almost completely negative. They did not seem to realise that they had had this effect on her.

It is important therefore to establish the right ground rules, so that people feel comfortable in exposing themselves.[10] It is vital to encourage group members to listen to and respect the views of others. This is especially relevant as clinical practice tends to be established as a set of black-and-white facts, an ethos which discourages divergence of opinion. Some writers have set out ways of ensuring that learning groups escape from such a bullying ethos by showing how divergence of opinion and debate can be codified as a proper part of the learning process of such groups.[10] Sometimes such disagreements or areas of doubt can be resolved by seeking out authoritative opinion, such as is provided by evidence based practice, but evidence based solutions are inappropriate or unavailable for many areas of practice.

Poor performance: failure to be involved in collaborative learning

In Chapter 8, Reed Bowden and John Schofield describe how many poorly performing doctors do not get involved in peer learning and have therefore cut themselves off from the great opportunity, which collaborative learning gives, for the critical renewal of practice. Small teams have fewer opportunities for informal collaborative learning, and ideally members of such teams should join multipractice learning groups.[10,14]

Poor performance: misguided one-on-one learning

In any team, however, and for all individuals at some time, collaborative learning can be an unhelpful and misguided process.

Two GPs were discussing the management of a particular cardiac condition, the discussion being initiated by a GP who had seen a case about which he felt puzzled. His colleague had the habit of speaking authoritatively. His opinions, on this occasion, were expressed with some authority, although he did admit that he wasn't certain. However, the enquiring GP felt that the authoritative GP had contributed some certainty to the situation and he acted accordingly. Later he did some private reading and discovered that neither of them had been right. Luckily the patient came to no harm.

Such a semi-fictional scenario represents the constant potential danger of collaborative learning – that of the blind leading the blind. I leave it to the reader to consider, from his or her own experience, how and why this happens and what can be done to minimise the risk. Do we need to be taught how to undertake such collaborative learning, so that the risks of misinformation are minimised? Do we already construct our own 'alarm systems' – safeguards against this happening? For example, why might the enquiring GP in the vignette above go on to double-check his facts through personal study – would he have his own personal alarm system? And how much do the advantages, especially to patients, of collaborative learning among health professionals outweigh its risks? These points are further discussed in Chapter 12.

Characteristics of personal learning

There are many characteristics of personal learning for health professionals in primary care. These are summarised in Box 3.3.

Box 3.3: Characteristics of personal learning

1   It should be sustainable and expedient.
2   It may be deliberate.
3   It may be experiential.
4   It may be stimulated by the responsibility of teaching others.
5   It relates to prior knowledge and prior training.
6   It relates to personal views and beliefs and experiences.

Sustainability and expedience

To sustain a lifetime of learning takes time. Working hours may be long; social and family life may be full. Some may feel that they do not have the time to do what they would like. Increasingly there is a movement towards protected time for learning within primary care teams. This is often achieved through the so-called shutdown sessions. In these the practice is able to shut down its services to patients for a few hours, diverting calls to the local GP co-operative, for example. Each of us has, however, a personal approach to how we undertake our personal learning, an approach built on habits and the circumstances of our lives.

Lifelong learning has to be sustainable within the pattern of each person's life. Over a professional lifetime of, perhaps, 30 years, each individual professional has to develop a comfortable and routine way of managing his/her learning needs, but one which is adaptable to changing circumstances. This nurse practitioner, whose children had long since left home, liked to use a quiet hour in the early morning to exercise her habits of disciplined learning.

> A nurse practitioner described how she read everything she could get her hands on. She said she read *Pulse*, *Doctor*, *GP*, *The Nursing Times*, *Practice Nursing*: she was an avid reader and read in her own time. She usually got up an hour early to do this – she had developed the discipline of a regular one-hour reading session.

How do health professionals in primary care approach their learning needs so that they can satisfy them easily? How do they manage to keep adding to their knowledge and skills? How do they maintain their working knowledge? Studies of GPs' reading habits have shown how little reading of the academic journals, such as the *BMJ*, is undertaken, and how much more widely the free press such as *Update* is read.[15,16] Such free journals contain excellent summary articles on how to manage common conditions in general practice, which are quick and easy to read. Easy access to knowledge is a major factor in whether professionals will bother to acquire such knowledge. On one multipractice based course, which took place in 1995 (before the Internet was available in surgeries), the health authority offered the 35 participants access to literature searches through its own authority based computers.[17] This meant making forward arrangements, followed by a round car journey of 32 miles: it represented a loss of two hours of working or leisure time. None of the participants availed themselves of this opportunity. It was too hard to arrange and too time-consuming. However, seven years later, in 2002, the situation has changed and the use of IT (from practice and home computers) for learning and accessing knowledge is much more widespread.

To accumulate knowledge and skills in an easy and sustainable way is not to act irresponsibly. Some methods of knowledge management are both quick and carry high levels of safety for patient care. One of the most commonly used is the seeking of expert opinion from colleagues, an approach which has already been described in the earlier part of this chapter in the section on collaborative learning.

A nurse practitioner described how he just went to the GP when he saw a dermatology condition he could not recognise – he called this '*seeking a second opinion*'.

A practice manager describes how she finds the answer to something she doesn't know:

> Question: What would you do to find out something that you don't know anything about?
> Answer: I would probably start off with another practice manager.

Here is an account from a GP describing a variety of ways in which she uses or has used colleagues to help her:

> A GP reported how most of her learning was from working experience. '*I think that most of what I know now, I've learned by experience.*' She knew where to find the answer. She was now able to admit when she didn't know and find out where the answer might be. So although as a new GP she hadn't known then what she knew now as an experienced GP, she could see how she had learned by experience along the way. This included learning through experienced colleagues. In her first practice, experienced colleagues had shown her how to do various techniques that she didn't know how to do, in terms of minor surgery and things like that. She felt that in terms of up-to-date practice, things moved on so quickly that at times she hasn't really the slightest clue what some of the hospital letters mean when they arrive at the practice. But she agreed that sometimes it didn't matter that she didn't know. At other times, however, she needed to know and she had various approaches to making sure she did understand things. She thought it was a question of trying to find out – to know where to go to find the information. She had no problem now picking up the phone and asking to speak to a consultant who had written her a letter that she didn't understand. She could say, 'I'm afraid I have no knowledge of this – can you run it past me? What do I need to know for this patient?' She thought that when she had first qualified, she had felt that she should know these things. It had only been with the passage of time that she had realised that she couldn't possibly know everything because there is just too much to know. It was more a process of recognising when she needed to find out more and having ways of doing so.

Deliberate learning

In Chapter 1 we referred to the place of both experiential and deliberate learning in WBL. Deliberate learning is helpful for the establishment of new roles in the practice setting and to overcome radical deficiencies in preparedness for the work. Primary care nurses have especially established their new roles (for example, in women's health and chronic disease management) through deliberate learning strategies, the majority going on certificated courses, some of which even require certificated updates.

GPs and nurses often describe their initial training as not preparing them for their present work. Nurses explained how their working experience as nurses, before entering practice nursing, had not prepared them at all for their new work. One nurse described how she had felt 'absolutely shocked ... and out of my depth completely' in her first week in the general practice setting.[1]

The hospital setting in which doctors and nurses train is different from the community setting in which they later work. The following type of statement is common: this from a GP.[1]

The skills we developed at medical school were largely reflected from our hospital work. The patients you see in general practice are different . . .

As there is no tradition yet of training nurses for general practice in the way that GPs are trained through vocational training, nurses most often achieve a new role for their general practice work through a progression of courses – for example, in chronic disease management and women's and children's health. This is a good example of the importance of deliberate learning in overcoming the initial non-preparedness for practice. As nurses undergo training for nurse practitioner status, receptionists are trained for healthcare assistant status and GPs train to gain specialist skills, such deliberate learning will become more common.

Deliberate learning: the role of practice based learning

As has been described earlier in this chapter, practice based learning has a role to play in deliberate learning. Practices may plan programmes of practice based learning which are well thought through and which contribute to significant advances in the work capacity of individuals. Such learning may integrate deliberate learning undertaken outside the practice (for example, by one member of the team) into new ways of working for the whole team.

Some of what benefits patients depends on the way in which the practice team organises care. Organising care is often a more important influence on improvements to patient care than on what one person knows or can do. Some personal learning, therefore, is about awareness of practice systems, and, as it were, the capacity of the team and all its individual members to work with both new knowledge and new systems.

Experiential learning

However, once having established a level of expertise and competence, there is no time to think that the rest will be plain sailing. The ever-changing nature of knowledge, the changing roles of primary care professionals and the changing expectations of how professionals will perform means that primary care professionals are never fully prepared.

Adjustments to pre-existing knowledge and skills occur in the main through experiential learning. The majority of these adjustments occur through the learning methods already discussed in previous paragraphs: reading, use of the computer for learning, reacting to work experiences, discussions with peer and expert colleagues. One of the skills is to know when one's present knowledge or skill level is inadequate and to be able to take appropriate action. Learning opportunities arrive daily and unexpectedly. Solutions to individual puzzlement are not only about academic knowledge: they are about satisfying the need to be competent and the need to act safely and wisely, in the patient's interest.

So, experiential learning is not just about learning about illnesses. It is also about learning to make judgements, to work safely, to work responsibly. This may mean knowing the rules about issuing certificates or about accessing benefits. This means being able to respect the patient's capacities and wishes. This means recognising the complexity of the technical and scientific part of work – being *au fait* with current knowledge and using it for the patient's benefit.

An elderly lady of 89 attended her GP with several complaints. One of these was the recent loss of vision in the left eye. The GP recognised his limitations in ophthalmology and asked her to attend the community optometrist in town. The optometrist's examination revealed that the condition was caused by vitreous floaters and that there was no evidence of a more serious condition, such as a detachment. The optometrist, however and for safety's sake, recommended to the GP that the patient be referred on to hospital. But the patient, being almost 90 years of age, was hesitant about a trip to the local hospital and preferred not to go unless it was really necessary. The GP phoned the hospital for further advice and spoke to a hospital doctor who reassured the GP that the patient could be managed through a watchful waiting policy and the condition was not serious in itself. He spelled out to the GP the actual symptoms that the patient might experience should a more serious situation such as detachment intervene. The GP was able to telephone the patient and reassure her that she need not at present go to hospital. He arranged follow-up with himself and let her know what to watch out for. He recorded the hospital doctor's telephone advice so other professionals in the practice were also aware of it.

Teachers as learners

The responsibility of teaching others

Many primary care health professionals are involved in teaching. Unlike those for whom teaching is a sole occupation, the primary care professional who teaches is firstly a practice manager or nurse or doctor. Teaching is usually a part-time occupation, perhaps done for only part of the week or sporadically to do with various projects. To be a teacher is to add something extra to professional practice. It is known that teaching is good for enthusiasm and good for keeping up to date. Teaching is listed in Chapter 12 as one of the methods for assessing one's own knowledge. Practices involved in teaching are also known to have higher scores on a range of organisational and performance quality indicators.[18,19] Many people relate how teaching ensures that you really understand something deeply enough so that you are able to give a convincing account of it to your student. A recently qualified student can act as a stimulus to an older colleague whose knowledge of the latest science is rusty.

Here is a practice manager explaining how she is training two new practice managers on other practices.[1]

Interviewer: *Okay, we'll carry on. Now you're a consultant. Now who's asked you to do that? The health authority?*

PM: *No, two different GP practices. They just asked me to go in and be their consultant.*

Interviewer: *Is this because they have two new practice managers, to help them get used to their job?*

PM: *Yes, the one in H has a new practice manager so she comes here about once a month and I go through what she needs to do and I'm doing appraisals with her from next week and I'm appraising her, appraising the staff. So that's kind of an ongoing training. And the one that I do in E ... I am monitoring her, as well, and teaching her, so I do that and I also do quite a lot of staff training and I do work with PCT when I'm asked.*

Interviewer: *What do you think the effect of all this is on your own learning?*

PM: *I think it's good because it makes you think about your own knowledge, because you have to check that you've got it right (laugh).*

Interviewer: *Yes, because you can be flying by the seat of your pants.*

PM: *Yes.*

Interviewer: *Somebody's depending on you to have it right.*

PM: *Exactly, so you have to double-check your facts. So it's good in that respect, it makes you check that you know what you're talking about. It also makes you look at how you deliver your information – because you know it, you've got a habit of assuming everybody else knows it and so it makes you stop and think, well, if I say this, do they know exactly what I mean? So it makes you question the people that you are actually teaching to make sure that they've got the right information from you. Because sometimes, you know, you think you've given the message and you haven't given the correct message. So it's made me look at the way I deliver it.*

To teach is to make sure that you are sure. Equally, to be a good teacher is to expose your capacity to work from uncertainty and to help others to share in the journey from not knowing to knowing better. This process is described in greater detail in the next section.

Teaching and learning: the admission of ignorance and the pursuit of inquisitiveness

Chapter 2 has already described the role of teaching in creating a certain type of excellence in a practice team. The activity of teaching, if it is work based, adds something extra to the working-learning team.

It would be wrong to assume that teaching only consists of imparting to others one's expertise, although this is a large part of it. In primary care teams, teachers are sometimes, and in some areas, ignorant or less knowledgeable than those whom they are teaching. Or they may have arrived at that place of wisdom where they can admit to their daily 'not knowingness'.

By saying this, I am suggesting that teachers should be committed to the journey of learning. Teaching should involve the capacity to communicate one's own commitment to be in 'constant learning mode'.

In Chapter 2, we also referred to Senge's writing on the learning organisation.[20] Senge writes about what he calls personal mastery, a characteristic which combines deep inquisitiveness with the willingness to admit to self and others ignorance and not knowing.

Personal mastery is not something you possess. It is a process. It is a lifelong discipline. People with a high level of personal mastery are acutely aware of their ignorance, their incompetence, their growth areas. And they are deeply self-confident. Paradoxical? Only for those who do not see that 'the journey is the reward'.[20]

Personal mastery is a quality that ensures an openness to constant learning: it is also a quality which, if possessed by one member of a team, can communicate itself to others. It may spread by contagion.

One GP who was interviewed spoke of her admiration for a partner who seemed 'open', inquisitive and able to admit his not knowing – he had the ability to use this as a stimulus for a shared enquiry between professionals.

Morton-Cooper and Palmer, in writing of learning support for new nurses, speak of the need to help practitioners articulate their uncertainty and lack of knowledge without fear of being seen as weak or helpless.[21] Dealing with uncertainty is tackled again in Chapters 7 and 12 of this book. Working colleagues who can show that vulnerability and uncertainty are part and parcel of the professional role act as teachers in the workplace – teachers not of fact but of a style of working and a way of surviving.

Present and previous experiences, present beliefs

In his book *Doctors on the Edge*, Linden West has described at length the way in which doctors have learned to distrust their personal stories.[3] He says:

> *Stories, as anthropologists remind us, are the means by which humans make sense of experience. It may be a big story, such as science, or a more personal one, as we seek to make meaning, for instance, from birth or death or illness. The difficulty is that doctors have been taught to distrust their personal stories in the name of big science. Such science can be a normalising truth that tends to disqualify, limit, deny or contain other potential stories . . . The problem is that of the profound split between personhood and medical practice.*

It is clear that doctors, nurses and practice managers have come to their professional practice with a variety of experiences in their personal lives.[1] They understand how these have significantly affected their practice.

Some of these experiences have been emotionally negative. For example, one GP described how she felt in awe of the 'able partners' in the group practice she had joined, and felt that this was inhibiting her.[1] She certainly did not feel able to ask for the support she needed. And when it came to the GPs sitting together to plan their own personal development plans, the lack of safety and structure effectively meant that no useful dialogue was achieved.

Some events in the professionals' lives had freed them up, and other experiences that might have been emotionally negative at one point in the individual's life had been turned into opportunities for personal growth and development. For example, the experience of illness in self or the family had stimulated them to learn more or helped them to empathise with the patients for whom they bore responsibility.

Personality and life experiences

Beliefs and life events can have a great effect on strategies for learning. Some practitioners have understood how earlier life experiences had helped to make them the sort of person they were, and how learning continued to contribute to that self-image.

Here is a nurse practitioner explaining his disciplined approach to self-advancement.[1]

> Interviewer: *... and yet you have had a whole new career. You've done such a lot with it.*
>
> NP: *Well, probably, I think it comes from my background and having to fight for confidence, as it were.*

And a GP:[1]

> I think that a lot of the people skills that I had or have now I actually learned not inside the medical course, because I did other things before I did medicine. I'd already learned how to talk to lots of different types of people from different walks of life, which is another skill you need for general practice ... to be able to get onto people's wavelengths ... We had no teaching on communication or how to go about having a consultation or anything like ... I don't really feel I was taught that as such. I feel that was more experience of life really.

Balancing the advance of a career against family responsibilities is another theme. A practice manager had almost finished a law degree at the age of 48, which had taught her an enormous amount that was useful for her role in primary care. And yet she had had to wait until she was nearly 50 to get this far, because of her earlier responsibilities as a mother.[1]

> PM: *I didn't really go to university until I felt my children were old enough that I didn't need to be there in the evening. So I postponed my university for 14 years to four years ago.*
>
> Interviewer: *Is that something (the delay) that you regret?*
>
> PM: *I felt okay that that held me back for 14 years because that's what I chose ...*

Learning from the personal experience of illness

Illness in family or self can be a stimulus to learning. It can also be a force for making the professional more understanding of his or her patients. This area is also covered in Chapter 7. One senior practice nurse related how her son had developed asthma and how the experience made her realise how she knew too little about asthma.[1] She then went on:

> *One thing, well there's two, but the one main one that influenced my need to learn if you like in nursing was my son developing asthma. I then realised my basic training was nowhere near enough. It didn't cover where I needed to know and that drove me to do the original asthma course.*

A GP related how the experiences of backache had taught her a lot, including greater sympathy for fellow sufferers.[1]

> *A lot of personal things have had a big influence, like I was getting a lot of back pain last year so I've gone to see a physiotherapist for the first time and I thought that was really nice to learn what she was doing; it makes me much more sympathetic to people with back pain. It makes me realise what you do every minute of the day affects it and how difficult it is to change what you do, so I use that as a way of learning something . . .*

Personal beliefs

Professionals come to their work with different beliefs about what makes a good doctor, nurse or manager. For some professionals, their view of good practice is to excel in the technico-scientific side of the work. For example, they see the primacy of audit and clinical governance in improving quality of care. For others, good practice is to do with other aspects of care, such as how the professional–patient relationship can promote healing. These varying beliefs do seem to affect strongly the way that individuals set about their learning.

Here is a GP who has an interest in the healing process, an interest which affects her choices about learning.[1]

> *GP: No, it's sort of a personal development thing for me that I'm going to do. I think one of the people going to it is one of the people who's learned a lot from some of the native American Indians. It is about how they do their healing and how they pick up needs within themselves and how they go about living healthy lives. I thought that might give me something different to think about and a different slant on things. I'm quite interested in alternative, so-called, medicine or ways of health and healing from other cultures, although I don't know very much about it. I'm quite interested because western medicine is really quite different for example from eastern medicine. And yet they're all living their lives and we're all living our lives but we're all approaching it in a completely different way. And I'm really interested in a more global way of healing if you like. What it is we do, that is ultimately healing or not. I mean, I have to get bogged down in HbA1cs and things as we all do.*

Interviewer: *But it's very important, all of that, isn't it?*

GP: *What, HbA1cs (laugh)?*

Interviewer: *No, what you just said about the role of the doctor as a healer.*

GP: *I'm more interested in that really. I learn the other things as I need them in the course of my work but I know a lot of the things that are good that take place in consultation would be very hard to audit in a tick box. And it's that more nebulous part of what goes on in a healing consultation that I'm more interested in really than if somebody's blood sugar is 12 or 10. But that's just an interest of mine.*

For others, the quality agenda is a major influence on learning and practice and they believe in this agenda.

Interviewer: *Yes, well the role, such as how does it influence your learning now that you know that you are governed by certain things? Like you must do audit and . . .*

NP: *I think it shows actually how you practise. You might think you practise in a certain way and do a certain thing but actually with audit in particular what is actually going on, it's written in black and white. So there is no sort of, oh yes everybody's on aspirin or whatever. Actually they're not, you know, only 60%. You know it's there so we can actually see what's going on in practice and hopefully alter that . . .*

And later:

Interviewer: *Okay, so let's say the results of audit of disease management schedules. What's the, what is that kind of influence on your practice?*

NP: *Yes, it does make you more thorough. And I think by being more thorough you are probably ultimately giving patients better care which is why we're here, so hopefully that's what's coming out of it.*

Life events and present and past experiences and beliefs have a great influence on personal learning. It is important to understand that individuals come to their jobs with a wide range of experiences, some of which are holding them back and some of which have been turned into opportunities for personal growth. Different individuals have different interests and beliefs. These may or may not be in line with the prevailing discourse in healthcare. For example, in the age of evidence based medicine it has become less fashionable to be interested in the art of healing. These are, of course, not either/or situations, because individuals have to try to integrate personal interests into the broader context of their work.

Discordancies of personal learning

Personal learning as described in this chapter is, to a large extent, reactive. One of the tasks, then, of personal learning is to develop a sense of awareness of what one's learning needs are and a sense of responsibility towards the task of learning. This process is described as the assessment of learning needs. We all have to say: '*I have discovered I don't know this very well or I can't do this very well – therefore I must remedy the situation.*' There are now new approaches towards professional learning – portfolios for nurses and professional development plans for GPs. This should mean that personal learning will be undertaken with a new sense of purpose and responsibility. The prediction must be that learning will become more purposeful and fewer learning opportunities will be neglected.

Richard Eve has already shown that different GPs differ widely in the frequency with which they identify learning needs from ordinary surgery based encounters.[22] Does this reflect different levels of neuroticism, with the more worried GPs finding more gaps in their performance, or are the GPs who report fewer learning needs unaware, over-defended or easily satisfied? We do not know the answers to these questions. Variation between individuals' biographies and beliefs also influences how, when and what is learned.

Some of the motivation for learning comes from personal experience and interest: in the public world, the personal and the affective aspects of learning are little valued. This is a difficult area because, plainly, what happens to professionals in their lives, what their beliefs and values are – all these are matters outside the service-led agenda, but these factors make a significant contribution to motivation and dedication. Rightly and practically, the service agenda has an enormous and powerful influence on learners. Professional practice will increasingly be judged by efficiency in attaining outcomes in prescribed areas, but motivations will remain part-grounded in the personal.

Conclusion

This chapter has discussed how professionals in primary care learn at present and what influences their learning. WBL is obviously central to collaborative and personal learning. In this book we define WBL as learning that takes place at work or, if it occurs elsewhere, is harnessed to the purpose of work. Collaborative learning is defined as learning which takes place through joint enquiry involving two or more people. Personal learning is defined as learning which meets individuals' learning needs. The different modalities of learning are discussed – whether the learning is undertaken formally or informally, whether by reading, use of IT and so on. Much learning is experiential: it occurs in response to the need for immediate help in various situations at work. Other

---

Box 3.4: Strategies for making collaborative and personal learning more effective

1 Make personal and collaborative learning more organised, disciplined and systematic.
2 Make sure that personal learning is integrated into the development of each practice, where this is appropriate.
3 Recognise your limitations and those of others.
4 Support yourself by being sensible and others by understanding more about their attitudes to practice and what motivates them.

---

learning is more deliberate. Professionals may take courses of training so that they can bring new skills to the practice – or such deliberate learning can occur during practice based learning sessions. Personal experiences affect our behaviour as learners, can be great teachers and can alert the professional to his or her need for further learning. Personal beliefs about the purpose of professional practice have a considerable influence on attitudes to learning. Practice teams differ in their capacity for pulling together all these different strands.

What, then, might be the ways in which health professionals can make their collaborative and personal learning more effective, more sophisticated, but keep it sustainable? A summary of ideas is included in Box 3.4. To start with, a sensible ambition would be to make personal and collaborative learning more organised, disciplined and systematic – for some people more of the same thing and for others a lot more. Another ambition should be to make sure that personal learning is integrated into the development of each practice, where this is appropriate. Collective work with others – whether individuals or teams – is an important stimulus to change, and the perception of 'falling behind' can stimulate extra effort, both in learning and in how work is organised. However, to the contrary, the feelings that surround the opportunities for learning can also be negative and inhibitory. The broader experiences of life do contribute to what is learned and how learning is undertaken. Personal interests and beliefs are strongly involved in attitudes to practice and learning. Just as duties to patients should be measured against the capacity to deliver these duties, so learning should be undertaken in a way which is sustainable. This rule should apply both to individuals and to teams.

Further reading

The Journal of the Learning Workplace can be accessed through www.tlw.org.uk.

References

1 Burton J and Perkins J (2003) *Accounts of Personal Learning from Primary Care.* (www.londondeanery.ac.uk/gp/home.htm)

2 Debreczeny S (2002) *Review of PCG Attached Primary Care Tutors.* (www.londondeanery.ac.uk/gp/home.htm)

3 West L (2001) *Doctors on the Edge.* Free Association Books, London.

4 Thomas D (2002) Tackling drug problems head on. *Medeconomics.* **November**: 28–30.

5 Chief Medical Officer (1998) *A Review of Continuing Professional Development in General Practice.* Department of Health, London.

6 Staley M (2001) Evaluating an in-house educational programme. *J Learning Workplace.* **3**: 12–16. (www.tlw.org.uk)

7 Burton J and Launer J (2003) *Supervision and Support in Primary Care.* Radcliffe Medical Press, Oxford.

8 Joiner R, Littleton K, Faulkner D *et al.* (2000) *Rethinking Collaborative Learning.* Free Association Books, London.

9 Bennis W and Biederman P (1997) *Organizing Genius. The secrets of creative collaboration.* Addison-Wesley, Reading, MA.

10 Hiew S, Sivananthan N and Burton J (2003) Self directed learning groups. In: J Burton and J Launer (eds) *Supervision and Support in Primary Care.* Radcliffe Medical Press, Oxford.

11 Peloso P and Stakiw K (2000) Small group learning format for continuing medical education. *J Continuing Med Ed in the Health Professions.* **20**: 27–32.

12 Thomas M (2002) PPDP: a tool for learning. First published in *Update*, 20 December 2001. Available in full in the 2002 volume of *J Learning Workplace*. www.tlw.org.uk.

13 Spurrell M (1999) Consultant learning groups in psychiatry: report on a pilot study. *Psychiatric Bulletin.* **24(10)**: 390–2.

14 Burton J (1998) Multipractice, self-directed learning groups in North Thames East region. *Ed Gen Pract.* **9**: 184–8.

15 Pitts J (2000) Reading habits of general practitioners within a primary care group. *Ed Gen Pract.* **11**: 175–8.

16 Allery L, Owen P and Robling M (1997) Why general practitioners and consultants change their clinical practice: a critical incident study. *BMJ.* **314**: 870–4.

17 Burton J (2000) Multipractice and interprofessional learning in the community: a problem based approach to improving cancer care. *Ed Gen Pract.* **11**: 51–7.

18 Ahmed S and Epstein L (2002) Would you make a good teacher? *Update.* **28 February**: 258–60.

19 Gray RW, Carter YH, Hull SA *et al.* (2001) Characteristics of general practices involved in undergraduate medical teaching. *Br J Gen Pract.* **51**: 371–4.

20 Senge PM (1992) *The Fifth Discipline – the art and practice of the learning organisation.* Century Business, London.

21 Morton-Cooper A and Palmer A (2000) *Mentorship, Preceptorship and Clinical Supervision.* Blackwell Science, Oxford.

22 Eve R (2000) Learning with PUNs and DENs – a method for determining educational needs and the evaluation of its use in primary care. *Ed Gen Pract.* **11**: 73–9.

CHAPTER 4

Work based learning and information technology

Jonathan Burton and Neil Jackson

A world with vast quantities of information without discerning judgement as to its worth is a world without knowledge.[1]

The importance of information technology in the National Health Service

In earlier chapters we have already described the importance of information technology (IT) in the development of the NHS and in the pursuit of personal and team learning. Key to the whole process is that individuals should have a basic competency in the use of IT.

In the Introduction, we described the UK government strategy in respect of the development of a patient-centred NHS and lifelong learning for the staff who serve patients. IT is central to the development of the NHS. The NHS plan emphasised the need to establish modern IT systems in every GP surgery with appropriate investment in NHS staff to develop and enhance IT skills. Prior to the publication of the NHS plan, the education, training and development strategy that supports the implementation of the NHS's national information strategy, *Information for Health*, had been launched in 1998.[2] This policy guidance was instrumental in setting out what needed to be done to develop new skills and changes in the culture of information management and use in the NHS. The strategy is basically intended to promote links with other policy initiatives in the NHS, e.g. continuing professional development, the NHS Learning Network and the NHS Leadership and Management Development Programmes. It also identifies roles and responsibilities for providing education and training in information management with account taken of local needs and the pace of change in the NHS, to be planned and delivered through Local

Implementation Strategies. Proficiency in the use of IT accrues from both opportunistic learning and deliberate learning.

In Chapter 3 we emphasised the importance of deliberate learning. Deliberate learning is an essential ingredient of WBL. It is the key element in the transition from the condition of 'no knowledge' to the condition of being fit for practice. Starting to learn about IT from scratch requires a deliberate approach, with a programme of formal teaching. The NHS recognises that some staff will need to undertake deliberate learning, in order to establish key skills in IT. To meet this challenge the NHS has adapted the European Computer Driving Licence (ECDL) as the reference standard for NHS staff.[3] The ECDL is an internationally recognised transferable qualification in seven key areas of competence (*see* Box 4.1).

Chapter 3 has described the flexible approaches to learning which health professionals use in order to learn opportunistically. Opportunistic learning builds on prior knowledge systems and occurs mainly in response to work based encounters and events. Opportunistic and incremental learning occurs, *par excellence*, in learning about IT. In many teams one or two individuals understand the primary care information system well and can help others in an ad hoc way to master particular tasks.

Box 4.1: The seven key areas of competence in computer use, as recognised by the European Computer Driving Licence (ECDL)

Each of the seven areas exists as a separate, stand-alone module.

- Basic concepts of IT.
- Using a computer and managing files.
- Word processing.
- Spreadsheets.
- Databases.
- Presentations.
- Information and communication.

The ECDL qualification is managed in the UK by the British Computer Society and most of the candidates complete the modules in one year, although the course can be extended over three years if required. The basic IT skills gained from undertaking the ECDL will enable healthcare professionals to access, for example, the National Electronic Library for Health, thus enabling an effective evidence based approach to working in the NHS.

Vignette 4.1: Printing a prescription
During the evening surgery session at a small rural practice, a GP, nurse and a new secretary-receptionist are on duty. Neither the nurse nor the secretary-receptionist knows how to line up the printer for printing off an urgent repeat prescription, although they have been taught to use the system for other tasks which they have to do routinely. The GP takes three minutes off between patients to show them how to do it.

In practice, once individuals gain a working knowledge of IT, most of their subsequent learning about IT is opportunistic and incremental. Such learning is driven by the need to use systems effectively enough to manage the daily requirements of working life.

The use of electronic information for learning

We write about this subject as practitioners and educators, drawing on our understanding of what is happening in the world of primary care at present. We are going to look at the two sources of electronic information which are most widely used in primary care. These are the Internet and primary care information systems. We use the term 'primary care information systems' to describe the dedicated computer systems that are used in general practice. The brief we have set ourselves is to discuss the strengths and limitations of these two sources of electronic information as a route for work based learning.

We will not be looking at the specialised, stand-alone programmes of computer-assisted learning (for example, in areas such as dermatology) and readers are referred to other authors for a fuller introductory description of these methods of learning.[4] The same authors discuss, in addition, the possibilities offered by web based approaches to certificated learning and the educational and support benefits of online virtual communities. The importance of these new approaches to IT-mediated learning is that, by not drawing practitioners away from their place of work, they satisfy some of the requirements for effective personal learning covered in Chapter 3 – expediency and sustainability, above all.

In our Introduction to this book we compared older forms of literacy, based on written text, with the newer forms which will be required in the computer age. Younie defines literacy as *how to read, create and analyse texts in order to participate in society*, and she contrasts the different cognitive functions required for accessing and reading printed text and accessing and making sense of electronic information.[1] She describes the new skills that will be required for this task under the broad definition of a flexible literacy. A flexible literacy includes having the right technical and computational skills to access information, being able to read it, make sense of it, critically analyse it, use it in a way which suits one's personal needs and then use it to participate appropriately in society.

Old-fashioned literacy prefers a linear logic, in which the reader goes from one point to another, as the writing is followed from beginning to end. The World Wide Web is organised in a non-linear way. Younie uses the adjectives multidimensional and dynamic to describe its organisation. It is known that many individuals prefer to print texts off the Web rather than read them online: this is partly to recreate the linear logic to which they have been accustomed since learning to read. Some of the resistance to the use of IT for learning rests in the difficulty that individuals experience in adapting to new forms of literacy. We will go on to show in this chapter how health professionals have already developed a flexible literacy in their approach to acquiring knowledge. They have already got a sense of how to use what is best out of what is available.

Information retrieval for work

On a daily basis, primary care health professionals need to check facts or establish some basic knowledge. The activity of seeking new knowledge or confirming old knowledge is known as information retrieval. When information is retrieved from an external source, such as a book or website, the user usually has no influence on its content. This content has been arranged by a third party. Most commonly, practitioners use textbooks and desk reference books such as the *British National Formulary* (*BNF*) for the purposes of information retrieval. But, sometimes this type of information is integrated into primary care information systems. *Mentor* is such a system and it is widely used. It is an online textbook attached to some primary care information systems, and is used like a paper textbook. Equally the *BNF* can be accessed online as the *e-BNF*.

The Internet is also used as an external source for data retrieval. Many health professionals use the Internet (either at home or at work) to search for health-related information. Patients increasingly use the Internet for this purpose and come armed with information from the Internet to their encounters with doctors and nurses.

> **Vignette 4.2:** The patient, the GP and various websites
> An elderly non-demented patient attended his GP with the question – how useful is ginkgo biloba for improving memory? The patient had read a website extolling its virtues and he wanted to know whether he should go on buying it at the health food store. The GP said he did not know. During the evening, at home, the GP decided to search the *BMJ* website via the Internet. The *BMJ* itself had no relevant literature, but the website gave the GP access to summaries of research in dozens of other journals. He chose *Evidence Based Mental Health* and found several summaries of articles in which the role of ginkgo biloba in dementia or cognitive decline was reviewed. After this 15-minute search he felt better prepared should he be posed a similar question later.

Another approach is to retrieve information from an internal source. An internal source of information is one that has been established and maintained by the users, in this case by the health professional or his/her team. The users control the content of the data. So, data about patients is created on the primary care information system through the process of recording aspects of the patients' health or ill health. This data acts a source of information for audit and other methods of quality control. The primary care information system is therefore, in part, a closed and controlled world of data about patients, created by the members of the team. But it also holds externally derived information, which can be used in conjunction with patient encounters.

The spread of the Internet

Nothing is changing faster than IT. Radio had to exist for 38 years before it could claim 50 million listeners worldwide. Television existed for 13 years before it reached the same target. The Internet was only created in 1994, but by 1998 it had 50 million users. By 2007, 13 years after its development, it is estimated that one third of the world's population will have access to the Internet.[5] This powerful tool is destined to change the way we access information and will have a profound effect on healthcare worldwide. We cannot, in the end, resist it and it will have an increasing influence on the way we learn. What resistance we offer is ritualistic, as James Gleick has described.[6]

So we engage in this ritual – the never ending, reluctant dance with the invader. Technology encroaches and we resist. Our resistance is sensible and honorable. And then later, we give up. In this case we connect.

The limitations of the Internet

The Internet as a source of information can be useful, but it may be no more useful than other sources of information. In fact, it may not only be no more useful, it may also take an inordinate amount of time to use. Experienced practitioners know how to access information from a variety of sources and many will discard an Internet search if it is getting nowhere or taking too long.

Vignette 4.3: The practice nurse, rabies vaccine and knowing where to go for information
A practice nurse was asked whether there was any latitude in respect of the BNF's advice on rabies vaccination and the length of time immunity would be established following primary vaccination and booster vaccination. She

wanted to be certain. She searched the Internet for more detailed information than that contained in the *BNF*. The information she found on a general search under 'rabies vaccine' was no more detailed than the information she had read in the *BNF*. The search, however, took her 15 minutes, while reading the *BNF* took 30 seconds.

As an experienced practice nurse, she knew that the next step was to telephone the office of the manufacturer of rabies vaccine in the UK. A five-minute phone call gave her a wealth of useful guidance, including the important information that the guidance published in the *BNF* was correct but that, in practice, and for someone who had missed the booster deadlines, a longer period of immunity could usually be expected.

The Internet as a source of information can be unreliable. Users have to know how to find reliable information on the Internet. Leach and Moon[5] tell the story of the 14-year-old boy who reported to a teacher that the Holocaust never happened. Asked how he had come across that information, the boy answered that he had found it on a web page at Northwestern University. Leach and Moon go on to write that knowledge of the Internet should not be about knowing how to use Windows or Internet Explorer. It should start with knowing how to assess the worth and value of a website. Leach and Moon write from the perspective of school teaching. School-age users of the Internet are likely to be far more naïve about the content and reliability of information on the Internet than are adult users undertaking professional work. We believe that experienced practitioners in primary care have already developed skills in using various sources of information, and most have already discovered what source is best used in different circumstances. They know how to recognise the information which is unreliable. They also know that the Internet is but one source of information. They know that they are better off using other, more traditional sources of information in some situations.

The strengths of the Internet

The Internet opens up the world of knowledge to everyone. In the health setting, the Internet gives patients access to the sort of information that was only obtainable a few years ago by professionals. For professionals, reliable Internet sites are useful in a unique way for certain kinds of knowledge retrieval.

Vignette 4.4: Accessing information to help in resolving a complaint
Three GP partners had to prepare for a discussion with a patient who had made an informal complaint against them. This concerned the delay in diagnosing an ectopic pregnancy. They used a search of the *BMJ* website, and discovered a recent and comprehensive review article on ectopic pregnancy.

This article confirmed that the patient's presentation was extremely unusual and they were able to share this information with the patient and her husband. The complaint was resolved as a result of this discussion. Although the practice library had some books on women's health, none of these was up to date and none contained the detailed information which had been obtained, on this occasion, via the Internet.

For professional use, the Internet is more useful if carefully chosen websites are used. There are many advantages of the Internet over other forms of information. Reliable Internet based information is up to date, usually free at the point of access and easily searched. Textbooks cost money and may rapidly become out of date. Paper journals may provide more up-to-date information than textbooks but they have to be stored and there is no way of indexing the information in them.

Primary care information systems

As we have explained earlier in this chapter, primary care information systems are, in part, closed worlds of data based on encounters with patients. They also carry information from external sources, such as online textbooks, *Mentor*, already described, and decision-making programmes like *PRODIGY* (see below).

Ten years ago (1992), Shum detected the end of the beginning for the computerisation of general practice.[7] By that time 76% of practices had computer systems and a further 10% had them on order. Ten years after Shum described the end of the beginning, we might be tempted to predict that we have reached the beginning of the end, an end in which healthcare information is only recorded as electronic data and healthcare decisions are based on appropriate information derived from electronic data.

As Gillies writes, it might be possible to demand that decision making should no longer be dependent on individual knowledge, memory and experience, because, as he says, *it is impossible for a generalist to know about it all.*[8] Examples of decision support[9] are shown in Box 4.2. Gillies argues that, because of the limitations of human capacity, information has to be made available and clinicians have to be encouraged to access it. *PRODIGY* (*see* Box 4.2) is the most widely used primary care based system designed to help with decision making. It steers individuals down decision-making pathways. Gillies is unsure how widely it is used nor how useful it has proved to those that do use it. This point is made by many GPs who use *PRODIGY*, and who recognise that, at present, decision support systems have their limitations.[10]

Not all encounters with patients are quantifiable – in fact, the majority are probably not. Primary care professionals tend to choose only to do what seems to be working well. Earlier in this book we have shown how work based

---

Box 4.2: Decision support systems[9]

CAS – Clinical Assessment System. This is the NHS Direct system. It uses a yes/no answer system until a conclusion is reached. Not suitable for general practice, where a range of clinical skills (often called soft skills) are used in making decisions about diagnosis and management.

PRODIGY – Prescribing RatiOnally with Decision support In General practice studY. Helps with decisions about prescribing after a diagnosis has been made. Makes the evidence clear on which suggestions are based.

Isabel – named after a child called Isabel who almost died after a rare complication of a common disease. This system is designed to show the range of possible diagnoses based on the symptoms and signs.

Dermis – a step-by-step system for identifying probabilities in dermatological diagnosis.

---

learning has to be able to be undertaken expediently and in a sustainable way – such are the demands on health professionals' time. All the evidence is that healthcare professionals will use electronic information systems in a way that suits them. They will record such information electronically that is useful for the care of patients and the efficient running of practices. They will disregard information or systems that are impenetrable or a waste of time.

Take the Read codes. These are the alphanumeric codes that were allocated by Dr Read to measurable aspects of healthcare. It is almost impossible to use Read codes for recording diagnostic data for each and every consultation, including the many patients who present with difficult-to-quantify complaints. Some practices may be doing this in a carefully thought-out way and as a part of research activity. But for others – is it worth it? No, because Read codes are too clumsy for recording the everyday, often non-disease, ailments that present in primary care.[11] On the other hand, almost all practices will have a policy to use Read codes for recording information on major illnesses. Such information can be used for audits of common chronic diseases. And audits that record aspects of care of, for example, hypertension are tools of inestimable importance in improving the care of the practice's population of patients with hypertension.

Just 15 years ago, when there was no electronic data of this nature, it was a really hard job to undertake a review of hypertension care. It could be done, in a sort of way, using various paper systems, but it was a tremendous sweat. When the time came, a year later, to repeat the review, another tremendous sweat ensued as a new search of paper records was mounted. Practice information systems have meant that this type of year-on-year audit is immeasurably easier to perform. Chapters 2 and 10 in this book set out how such records of performance form the basis of much practice development planning and the learning or activity that needs to go with it.

Vignette 4.5: Action to show whether care of patients was improving or not

In a year-on-year audit of the care of patients with diabetes, a practice failed to achieve the standards it had set itself. In particular, few patients were recorded as having had an annual eye examination. Most of the patients were having eye checks, which were being undertaken by local community optometrists in the city. They, in turn, sent copies of their findings to the practice. But these were not being recorded on the practice information system in a searchable way. This problem was tackled at one of the practice's regular educational meetings and the practice manager arranged for a member of the clerical team to routinely enter details of the annual eye check onto a searchable template within the practice information system.

Summary

Information technology is vital for the development of the NHS and the UK government has developed strategies to ensure that it becomes well established. Health professionals in primary care first need to establish basic competence in the use of IT. After this, most subsequent learning about IT is opportunistic. A new sort of literacy is required for using the Internet for WBL – a literacy which is adapted to the non-linearity of information on the Internet, and which is capable of judging the value and worth of particular Internet sites. Patients use the Internet more and more and health professionals often need to 'work up' subjects and questions which patients have brought to them from the Internet. Practice information systems can carry online textbooks and decision-making programmes. The former are the equivalent of paper textbooks, and the latter are of some but limited use at present. The main use of practice information systems for work based learning is in the field of audit and quality of care. Information retrieval may occur through use of IT but, often, is more easily achieved through use of textbooks or consulting with colleagues.

References

1   Younie S (2001) Developing a cognitively flexible literacy. In: M Leask (ed.) *Issues in Teaching Using ICT*. Routledge-Falmer, London.

2   Department of Health (1998) *Working Together with Health Information – a partnership strategy for education, training and development*. HMSO, London.

3   The European Computer Driving Licence (ECDL) website: www.ecdl.co.uk/nhs.

4 Jamieson A and Rennison T (2001) Information, learning and the new technologies. In: Y Carter and N Jackson (eds) *Guide to Education and Training for Primary Care*. Oxford University Press, Oxford.

5 Leach J and Moon B (2000) Pedagogy, information and communications technology and teachers' professional knowledge. *Curriculum Journal*. 11: 385–404.

6 Gleick J (2002) *What Just Happened*. Pantheon Books, New York.

7 Shum D (1992) The end of the beginning. *Br J Healthcare Computing*. 10: 24–5.

8 Gillies A (2002) *Providing Information for Health*. Radcliffe Medical Press, Oxford.

9 The Informatics Review website: www.informatics-review.com/decision-support.

10 Mimnagh C (2002) The systems that help GPs to heal. *GP*. **2 September**.

11 Launer J (2002) Read codes: taking the mickey or just a pain in the backside? *Doctor*. **22–29 August**.

CHAPTER 5

Apprenticeship systems and work based learning

Vicky Souster and Neil Jackson

By watching their elders the young people learned what they would soon be doing themselves and what they in turn would show their successors.
            (Pliny the Younger, c 62–c 113 AD. *Epistles*, viii, 14)

Introduction

This chapter is divided into four parts.

- Apprenticeship as a learning process.
- Modernising the principles of apprenticeship to enhance effective learning.
- Effective apprenticeship in the general practice setting.
- Conclusions.

In Europe there have always been two traditional methods of teaching and learning. Gear *et al.* describe the first as the didactic tradition, which can be traced down through the ages via monasteries, universities and schools.[1] The second is located mainly outside educational institutions:

It involves learning by doing, typically on the job, and the acquisition of knowledge and skill under the supervision of a more experienced practitioner, of whom one gradually becomes more independent. It is often self directed and relies heavily on oral communication. It is typically assessed in terms of competence or mastery of performance rather than through examinations.

Historically, the apprenticeship system of the medieval trade and craft guilds was a type of learning and teaching partnership that demonstrates all three criteria of work based learning. It was learning for work, at work and from work:

the practical skills of the craft or trade were learned only by the practice of that craft under close supervision from a master. Traditional ways of training doctors and nurses embraced these principles and working practices, including the acceptance of low pay and long hours in return for the privilege of learning from a master, who was the senior doctor or nurse supervising a small group of trainees. Even the tradition of apprentices living in their place of work was true of doctors and nurses until fairly recently, and some junior staff still live on site.

Modern students and teachers may dismiss apprenticeship as archaic and impractical, but this way of learning actually has a sound base in the theories that attempt to explain effective teaching and learning strategies. It is also a tradition that is alive and well in the general practice setting.

This chapter discusses the efficiency and effectiveness of apprenticeship as a form of work based learning, examines some examples of adaptation to the modern healthcare environment, and finally focuses down on vocational training for general practice by exploring the relationship between the GP trainer as a 'master' and the GP registrar as an 'apprentice'.

Apprenticeship as a learning process

Apprenticeship is not a passive way of learning. It can only be effective if the learner embraces the learning environment and decides to gain as much as possible from the day-to-day experience of work. Ramsden cites Bruner, who states that knowing is a process not a product. He goes on to state that *'learning is applying and modifying one's own ideas; it is something the student does, rather than something that is done to the student'*.[2] An awareness that one is on a journey towards skills and knowledge but will never actually reach the end is the essence of mastery. The best teachers are those who are continually learning themselves.

Those learning the craft of healthcare in a general practice setting need mentors and teachers who can model lifelong learning skills, and a passion to gain understanding, not just pass on knowledge or information. In GP training the setting allows for one-to-one training which is much harder to achieve in larger organisations. This year of close supervision allows GP registrars to gain clinical, organisational and professional understanding of their future role.

It is useful to examine what may be going on during this learning experience. Cheetham and Chivers suggest that there are two main processes in professional development: instruction and coaching.[3] Instruction is defined as *'the inculcation of specific knowledge or skill related principles to one or more individuals at the same time'*. Coaching is described as *'one to one learning support tailored to the needs of an individual'*. The authors draw on Bruner's metaphor of a coach as providing expert scaffolding to support the learner. Like real scaffolding, the support can be adjusted to the learners' needs, and dismantled when it is no longer needed. Gagne suggested that this can only happen when the conditions are suitable, and this is dependent upon the coach *directing the trainee's attention towards significant factors as well as imparting the hidden secrets of mastery*.

Why is this process so intimately linked to the workplace setting? The answer may be related to the insufficiency of language to convey certain principles. Without the language to describe them, there is no way that these things can be taught in a classroom or even a work based tutorial setting. The inability to describe the things that need to be learned was explored by Gamble in her study of apprentice cabinet makers in South Africa.[4]

Gamble studied a group of apprentices by observing them for two years. She found that the most important aspects of learning were never explicitly taught, but were the focus of the modelling process for the apprentice. The formal modules that the colleges produced did not influence the behaviour of the master – the master appeared to teach in a random or incidental fashion. In practice there was no intervention in the pupils' work unless they were in danger, or had a wrong body position. In the case of the latter, the master would take the wood and demonstrate the correct position and perform the movement. Drawing diagrams of the piece of furniture was the main means of communication between masters and apprentices. The quality of their work depended on them both being able to visualise a three-dimensional spatial arrangement, which no drawing can fully represent. Weak students were always described as those that couldn't draw.

When discussing this study with a young GP, she told me of points in her training when senior staff had taken her hands and put them in the right position so that she could feel something that the expert clinician had discovered in examining a patient. Doctors and cabinet makers both undergo formal preparatory training before their practical apprenticeship. Both learn about the spatial relationships between components of a three-dimensional object by looking at diagrams (in the doctor's case anatomy drawings and models). They cannot actually begin the real learning associated with their working lives until they are exposed to concrete examples of either three-dimensional furniture or three-dimensional bodies. At that point both have to make a leap of imagination in order to visualise what needs to be done with the concrete reality in front of them. For many healthcare practitioners (e.g. physiotherapists, nurses and doctors) this will also involve the skill of listening, and linking the patients' thoughts, feelings and perceptions to something which may (or may not) be happening in the body.

The critical aspect of mastery that was conveyed to successful apprentice cabinet makers was the *unity of thought and action, conception and execution, hand and mind*, in which *no distinction is made between "knowledge" and "skill"*.[4] It is interesting that in education for clinical staff these elements are commonly split up, and 'attitudes' are added for good measure.

The transmission of higher level skills could simply be explained as a result of the apprentice copying behaviour modelled by the master, but there is evidence that a rather more complex process is taking place. Cheetham and Chivers cite research by Bucher and Stelling which examined how professional trainees acquire 'professional identities'.[3] They disproved the theory that trainees model themselves on an individual mentor, and demonstrated that an amalgam of role models is used. They summarised five different types of role model: partial, where particular characteristics may be picked from different role models; charismatic, an idealised global model; stage, who demonstrate what to expect at a later stage in their career; option, models who provide examples of alternative career paths; and negative, role models who exhibit 'how not to be'. This work was supported by the research of Cheetham and Chivers, who reported that individuals who were influenced by role models '*had copied elements from a number of different people, rather than modelling themselves on any one person*'.[3] Only a few respondents out of the 452 participants in their study had modelled themselves on particular individuals. Several had been strongly influenced by negative role models who taught them 'how not to do things'.

The findings of Cheetham and Chivers regarding learning from experienced colleagues are pertinent to the subject of apprenticeship. Many interviewees described an '*almost unconscious absorption of skills through a form of osmosis*'.[3] There was no conscious effort to copy these colleagues, and they were not aware of closely observing them. Some felt that this had helped them to develop '"*know how*" *of a variety not easily articulated, as well as how to behave as a professional*'.[3] The authors note that the process has much in common with traditional apprenticeship learning. As well as working with more experienced colleagues the work of Cheetham and Chivers identified powerful learning experiences associated with teams and para-professionals, such as switching perspectives by working with people from different professional disciplines.

Modernising the principles of apprenticeship to enhance effective learning

Unlike the attitudes of master cabinet makers who would observe but rarely intervene, modern trainers are likely to provide support and care for learners, as well as encouraging them to reflect on their learning and why they are learning it. Learners may be encouraged to solve problems with suitable supervision, articulate their reasoning, and work in partnership with seniors to seek and respond to feedback about their performance. This model of instruction has been summarised in Box 5.1. The authors have also described the process as 'cognitive apprenticeship'.

> **Box 5.1:** Model of instruction based on Collins *et al.* (1989) cited by Cheetham and Chivers[3]
>
> The elements of instruction or 'cognitive apprenticeship'.
>
> 1 Modelling (by an expert).
> 2 Coaching (which the authors see as the learner practising while the coach offers feedback).
> 3 Scaffolding (the notion of providing support which is gradually reduced as the learner becomes more proficient).
> 4 Articulation (getting trainees to describe their reasoning or problem-solving processes).
> 5 Reflection (which the authors see as comparing their own reasoning or problem-solving processes with those of an expert or peer).
> 6 Exploration (where trainees take on problem solving without support).

Organisational changes in healthcare have transformed the learning environment and in many cases these changes have been welcomed. Some hospital consultants, however, are worried by the breakdown of traditional apprenticeship methods of learning for junior hospital doctors. They feel that the new shift systems and larger consultant teams have prevented junior doctors from forming strong supported relationships with senior staff. In fact the apprenticeship still continues, but with more junior staff such as senior registrars and senior house officers (SHOs). It remains to be seen whether the quality of the training will suffer as a result, but initial findings are that the smaller gap between the junior and senior positions enhances close supervision and provides a more comfortable, supportive relationship.

In an editorial by Bain (1996) the American Pew Health Services Commission (1993) was quoted as an example of how Britain should modernise its training for general practitioners.[5] The commission highlights the greatest danger in apprenticeship learning, the narrow focus that can restrict experience:

> *If specific educational outcomes are clear, the next step is to design the teaching and learning processes to reflect those outcomes. The apprenticeship model had many strengths but can result in a narrow focus as opposed to broadening the minds of these young doctors.*

Modernising educational practice sounds like an enormous task, especially if one takes into account changing the attitudes of some senior clinicians, but there is much that can be done and has been done successfully. The key is to consider the organisation of the educational experience, and to find ways in which young doctors can become partners in the learning rather than subjects of it. This may mean that the apprenticeship is not to a person, but to a team.

An interesting example of team apprenticeship was discovered during an unpublished research project by Souster and Marriott into innovative training posts set up and managed by the South London Organisation of Vocational Training Schemes (SLOVTS).[6] GPs in training worked in a community based post, where the mentoring was done by a team of specialist nurses. All six elements in the model of instruction proposed by Collins *et al.* were operating in this post, but the thing that the SHOs enjoyed most was the final stage of 'exploration', and this seemed to be a critical part of the learning process. It was the key factor in building confidence in new clinical skills, and was viewed by both the SHOs interviewed as the most enjoyable aspect of the training:

> *I suppose it was the independence and, for the first time really, the experience of being a doctor, um, on your own, making decisions (...) you really feel like you make a difference, which I'd never experienced before, having only worked in hospital.* (SHO)

Competence to this level of working was also built up by the modelling of a community consultant, but she was not present in the unit for the majority of the time. The SHOs reported that their most formative experience was the 'support' of the team of specialist nurses who actually manage the unit. This was provided during weekly case discussion meetings and one-to-one tutorials. The SHOs were encouraged to reflect on their clinical management, to articulate why these choices were made, and feedback was given about the doctor's performance. The specialist nurses were in fact providing coaching, scaffolding and the opportunity to explore new skills.

The SLOVTS research project also uncovered some aspects of the hospital environment that have been slow to change. Young doctors still feel nervous about challenging the practice or ideas of their seniors, because the environment is not conducive for them to do so. The idea of a partnership, where learning is an adventurous road travelled by both teacher and learner, is probably more common in the general practice setting than the hospital.

Many junior doctors and consultants still rely on traditional methods of learning (the ward round, the lecture and the case presentation) to satisfy the requirements that the junior doctors' job is a training post. These things may well be very beneficial and sometimes are the most appropriate way to learn about certain subjects, but they perpetuate the idea that the junior doctor is not a partner in the learning process, but a recipient of it. In some cases they fail to provide what Janet Grant describes as a 'climate for learning'. This entails providing learners with a safe environment where they can reveal deficiencies and problems. Grant and Marsden identified positive attitudes of seniors to juniors as the key to this: '*Until juniors are allowed to fail, to not know, to ask questions openly and without scorn, a climate for learning cannot be created.*'[7]

For junior doctors aspiring to be 'masters' in general practice, apprenticeship to hospital specialists may be unhelpful. They do not wish to acquire mastery in the profession of the master, but need to master skills and knowledge that can be used in general practice later. This can be a confusing situation for the apprentice unless the 'master' has the skills to adapt the training to suit the real needs of the junior doctor. It is not easy for the junior doctor to manage, and the role of the course organiser (who is a GP) is critical. He or she has to broker an agreement between the consultant and the junior doctor, so that statutory training needs are met, personal learning needs are met and the junior doctors can provide a useful service to the hospital or department they are based in.

The traditional way of maintaining a general practice focus in hospital training posts involved the course organiser coming to assessment meetings with the junior doctor and the hospital consultant. Pressure on GPs' time has made it harder for them to extract themselves from surgery to attend these meetings. Also this formative assessment meeting happens halfway through the post, so much time may already have been wasted. An alternative approach is in place in south east London, which involves consultants and SHOs forming a joint learning agreement at the beginning of the training period. The junior doctors are encouraged to negotiate the educational process early on, and they are given clear objectives that guide them towards appropriate learning. It is much easier for them to plan their learning when there are clear boundaries to the extent of it. Having some objectives also helps them to identify which ones they have already met, or partly met, in other clinical situations, and provides a progress marker at the mid-point assessment.

Junior doctors are encouraged to be proactive at every stage, seizing appropriate learning opportunities as they arise and giving feedback on their own experience of the training process. The importance of the consultants in this process is, of course, paramount as they provide induction for new staff, negotiate the learning agreement with the GP trainee, provide clinical supervision and model expert professional behaviour for their own speciality.

Whatever structures are in place to support the learning process the most important support for learners comes from the consultant or other senior clinician who can provide supervision. This could be seen as an example of scaffolding and is critical to the learning experience. Without adequate supervision the junior doctors are left to make decisions that are outside of their competence, putting themselves and patients at risk. Another possible problem which prevents effective work based learning is that of reducing the doctors in training to observers, who are given no freedom to make clinical judgements, and therefore no responsibility. If new skills are not practised, they cannot be tested, and the senior cannot give clear feedback about performance. The SHO becomes a passive observer of experts. The most effective training, which was also the most enjoyable training, managed to strike a balance between freedom and supervision.

Effective apprenticeship in the general practice setting

This section of the chapter will be explored under five main headings.

- The GP trainer/trainee (GP registrar) relationship.
- The trainer as the teacher and master.
- The trainee (GP registrar) as the apprentice.
- Teaching styles.
- WBL and GP training.

The GP trainer/trainee (GP registrar) relationship

It has often been said that the relationship that exists between the GP trainer and GP trainee (registrar) is unique:

The most important factor in the educational process is the trainer/trainee relationship itself.[8]

Pereira Gray classified various models of relationships based on his discussions with a number of trainees on different GP vocational training schemes.[9] These are summarised as follows.

- *Real*:
  - employer/employee
  - doctor/patient.

- *Analogous*:
  - animal trainer
  - puppet on a string
  - driving instructor
  - military model
  - producer/actor
  - parent/child
  - older sibling
  - doctor/patient.

To this impressive list we can add master/apprentice. Here the GP trainer may be regarded as proficient or an expert in general practice, exhibiting the features of personal mastery. However, he or she must also have awareness of his or her personal strengths and weaknesses and a willingness to indulge in lifelong learning. The GP trainer will also recognise the connection between personal learning and organisational learning by a sustained commitment to developing his or her practice as a learning organisation.

On the other hand, the GP registrar, as the trainee or the apprentice, is a beginner or a novice learning the trade of general practice by being employed in the GP trainer's practice.

Although the influence of the GP trainer as a role model for the GP registrar is often profound, the very essence of the trainer/trainee relationship is the dynamic two-way educational process whereby the GP trainer can also learn from the GP registrar. This is particularly so when the registrar comes into the training practice fresh from the SHO part of training equipped with the knowledge of the latest advances in hospital medicine.

The trainer as the teacher and master

The Joint Committee on Postgraduate Training for General Practice (JCPTGP) in its publication *Recommendations on the Selection of General Practice Trainers* states that the greatest influence on GP registrars is the example presented by their trainers as doctors.[10]

In order to become an approved GP trainer in the United Kingdom general practitioners must reach the required standards as defined by the JCPTGP. The attributes or characteristics of the GP trainer are many and are classified under three main headings by the Joint Committee as follows.

- The trainer as a doctor: appropriate knowledge, skills and attitudes as a clinician.
- The trainer as a teacher: personal qualities, preparation for lecturing, organisation of teaching, teaching abilities, use of assessment methodology.
- The training practice: premises, staffing, record systems, library facilities/teaching aids, etc.

In terms of personal mastery the GP trainer must exhibit these attributes and demonstrate the required quality standards and it is hoped that the GP registrar as the apprentice will aspire to achieve these high levels of practice during the time spent in the training environment.

The trainee (GP registrar) as the apprentice

Roger Neighbour in his book entitled *The Inner Apprentice*[11] highlights the importance of the evolving relationship between teacher and pupil. He goes on to explain that the '*relationship of tutelage [between master and apprentice] is the*

*necessary extension of and framework for, the effective one-to-one teaching exempli-
fied by Socrates'*. The pivotal influence of this profound Greek philosopher (469–
399 BC) is referred to again later in this chapter in relation to teaching styles.

In relation to effective apprenticeship in the GP setting, however, what are
the educational needs of the GP registrar? How should the GP trainer and the
training system meet these educational needs? In this respect the 'one-to-one'
teaching relationship between trainer and registrar, while being crucial, is an
integral part of the registrar's overall educational programme during the time
spent in the training practice. This will include both regular tutorials in protected time and ad hoc teaching, e.g. around problem cases. The registrar's
needs must also be met by the provision of appropriate induction into the training practice; having a named educational supervisor to deputise in the absence
of the trainer; written educational aims for the training period; regular formative assessment of his or her educational needs linked to an educational plan;
protected release to the local GP vocational training scheme; access to the practice library and educational facilities; relevant study leave; training in clinical
audit and support with undertaking the summative assessment programme.

Teaching styles

In *The Future General Practitioner: learning and teaching*, the authors emphasise
that the teacher (or 'master') must have an awareness of what his or her trainee
(or 'apprentice') needs to learn.[12] Inherent to this is the competence of the teacher to help the trainee in identifying what is required to be learned and to stimulate the process of appropriate self-directed learning.

The authors go on to identify four teaching styles which maybe exhibited by
the GP trainer.

- *Authoritarian – To 'tell and sell'.*
  A domineering approach where facts are passed from trainer to trainee.
  Here the teacher may not encourage questioning by the trainee which
  could challenge his or her authority or 'mastership'.
- *Socratic – 'Teaching by question and answer'.*
  The teacher always asks and the trainee always answers. This in turns acts
  as a trigger for more questions and the teacher imparts new facts when the
  trainee (as the learner) demonstrates areas of deficiency or ignorance.
- *Heuristic – 'To find out for yourself'.*
  Encouraging the trainee to take responsibility for self-directed learning –
  that is to say 'learning by doing'.
- *Counselling.*
  A less directive style with the aim of encouraging the trainee to understand the interactions taking place between him/herself and the material
  being learned.

The ideal GP trainer should be an exponent of these different styles, which can be applied in a range of different situations. In practice, however, all GP trainers have strengths and weaknesses as teachers and therefore this may not be possible. The accomplished GP trainer will be aware of his or her weaknesses and will compensate for these by other means to the advantage of the trainee.

WBL and GP training

GP training in primary care takes place in a number of different settings in which the GP registrar will experience learning by a variety of different methods. These include learning from patients; learning from peers (other GP trainees, especially at the local vocational training scheme); learning from the GP trainer, his or her partners or consultant colleagues; learning from the multiprofessional practice team; learning from specific topics (for example, in the tutorial setting with the GP trainer); or learning independently through access to books, journals, articles and increasingly by electronic means/information technology.

Today's GP registrar is the GP of tomorrow and must be 'fit for the purpose' of surviving in the complex environment of the new NHS. Given this situation, it becomes necessary for additional learning to take place at the organisational level (e.g. primary care trusts) and in the wider context of the 'three systems of the NHS', i.e. service provision, education and training, and research and development.

Wherever learning takes place for the GP registrar, the principles of WBL can be applied and it is helpful in this context to recall our earlier definitions of WBL as given in this book, i.e. learning for work, learning at work and learning from work.

Learning for work

The tutorial between GP trainer and GP registrar may be defined in different ways but typically takes the form of face-to-face contact on a weekly basis in protected time. It may last for up to two hours, be topic based and directed towards ensuring that the registrar becomes clinically competent. The role of the trainer may vary in the tutorial according to the current needs of the registrar. In order to encourage learning for work the trainer, using a topic-based approach, might, for example, request the registrar in preparation for the tutorial to read around the subject of hypertension and its management in general practice.

Learning at work

Learning from the practice team at practice business or clinical meetings is an example of learning at work for the GP registrar. Practice staff, both medical and non-medical, play an important part in the registrar's learning and development during the GP training programme. Establishing good working relationships with the various members of the core practice team and the wider primary healthcare team (PHCT) is essential for the GP registrar. There is also much to be learned by 'sitting in' with each member of the team in the practice or observing PHCT healthcare professionals at work while undertaking home visits.

Learning from work

As is often the case in the GP registrar training programme, joint surgeries are conducted whereby both GP trainer and GP registrar consult together with patients. Between each consultation, discussion can take place between trainer and registrar about various issues relating to the patients seen, including effective history-taking and communication, preventive care, differential diagnosis of the patients' presenting complaint, appropriate investigation and further management, etc. Often these joint consultations may be videotaped and reviewed at a later date by permission of the patients concerned. This is a powerful learning experience in which the registrar's communications skills can be assessed and enhanced and the various models of the consultation can be explored. Both joint surgeries and videotaped consultations can be considered as effective examples of learning from work.

Conclusions

Work based learning in primary care involves learning in many spheres, including the clinical, the organisational, the personal and the interprofessional aspects of working life. The methods by which senior or experienced staff teach junior or inexperienced staff are clear, but the mechanism of transferring knowledge and experience is less well understood. Apprenticeship is a way of describing the 'osmosis' of these things from the teacher to the learner.

Recent educational theories have highlighted the importance of learners being aware of their status as learners and their need to optimise learning situations in everyday work. For learners, experiential learning, reflection on that learning, and awareness of cognitive and emotional 'blocks' to learning are now explicit in many training programmes. This raises their awareness of the factors which drive learning.

The idea of the single expert model, who trains and grooms a young practitioner in isolation, is now very out of date. Exposure to other role models (including those from other professions) and a more diverse learning experience is essential for staff in general practice. However, the primary attachment to a senior who can (ideally) build a relationship of trust and support to the learner, removing supportive 'scaffolding' when appropriate, seems to be a very popular and effective way of training staff. It transcends mentoring as it involves close observation and feedback regarding the novice's developing skills.

Primary care educators dealing with staff shortages and recruitment problems may find that this strategy provides an attractive alternative to college based professional training programmes for staff other than GPs. The appointing of 'masters' in practice management and nursing would affirm and reward skilled staff currently in post, and increase the number of teachers in the community. The apprentice could provide extra help to the practice, while learning the higher level of skills that characterise professionalism and mastery.

In every professional group, the most important relationship during the development of professional skills is that of working with a master in that profession. Even then, a wise modern 'master' will be aware that he or she can only provide part of the jigsaw puzzle of experience and teaching that young practitioners need. If mastery is separated from connotations of arrogance and control, and apprenticeship is divorced from its history of abuse, the relationship that still operates in GP training is an effective and important educational strategy.

References

1 Gear J, McIntosh A and Squires G (1994) *Informal Learning in the Professions*. Department of Education, University of Hull.

2 Ramsden P (1992) *Learning to Teach in Higher Education*. Routledge, London.

3 Cheetham G and Chivers G (2001) How professionals learn in practice: an investigation of informal learning amongst people working in professions. *J European Industrial Training*. **25(5)**: 248–92.

4 Gamble J (2001) Modelling the invisible: the pedagogy of craft apprenticeship. *Studies in Continuing Education*. **23(2)**: 185.

5 Bain J (1996) Vocational training: the end or the beginning? *Br J Gen Pract*. **46**: 328–30.

6 Souster V and Marriott P (2002) *Organising Education to Create a Climate for Learning. Research report*. SLOVTS, London (unpublished).

7 Grant J and Marsden P (1992) *Training Senior House Officers by Service Based Learning*. Joint Centre for Education in Medicine, London.

8 Stott P (1970) Learning general practice – the experience of one trainee. *Journal of the Royal College of General Practitioners*. **29**: 53–8.

9 Pereira Gray D (1982) *Training for General Practice*. Macdonald & Evans, London.

10 The Joint Committee on Postgraduate Training for General Practice (2001) *Recommendations on the Selection of General Practice Trainers*. JCPTGP, London.

11 Neighbour R (1992) *The Inner Apprentice*. Kluwer, Lancaster.

12 Royal College of General Practitioners (1972) *The Future General Practitioner: learning and teaching*. RCGP, London.

CHAPTER 6

Interprofessional issues and work based learning

Hugh Barr

Introduction

This chapter distinguishes between work-located and work-related learning. It employs the term 'work-located' when the learning occurs in the workplace and 'work-related' when the learning occurs in a college, training centre or elsewhere provided that it is designed explicitly to inform practice. Work-related learning is thereby distinguished from academic learning.

Similarities and differences are identified between work-located and work-related learning, differences that enable each to reinforce the other.

When does learning become interprofessional learning? When two or more professions learn from and about each other to improve collaboration and the quality of care for patients, if the definition commended by the UK Centre for the Advancement of Interprofessional Education (CAIPE) is adopted.[1] Defined thus, much of the learning described in this book is interprofessional.

Two thirds of 'initiatives' reported in successive UK surveys of interprofessional education can be described as work-located and only one third as work-related.[2,3]

Evidence from a systematic review shows how work-related interprofessional learning can, under favourable conditions, lay foundations for collaborative practice by enhancing mutual understanding and modifying perceptions, while work-located interprofessional learning can, again under favourable conditions, change practice by helping to resolve problems, implement policies and improve the quality of care.[4]

Conditions deemed favourable include institutional support, equality of status between learners, positive expectations, a co-operative learning atmosphere and attention to differences as well as similarities,[5] based upon the application of the 'contact hypothesis' originally formulated to address race relations' issues in the United States.[6] Satisfying those conditions in some work-related pro-grammes[7–10] is thought to account for progress in improving interprofessional relations, failure to satisfy them for lack of progress.[10,11] This carries implica-tions for work-located learning where effecting change and improvement depends upon establishing trust, mutual respect and give and take between the parties.

The remainder of the chapter offers some interprofessional perspectives on work-located and work-related learning, calling upon experience and examples from the literature and from other chapters, comparing and contrasting some of the many forms that interprofessional learning takes. It deals with continuing learning, but picks up some implications for pre-registration studies at the end.

Work-located learning

Earlier chapters contain examples of interprofessional learning. There was the nurse and GP who acknowledged their ignorance to each, consulted the rele-vant bulletin then shared their new-found knowledge with colleagues, which reinforced their collective learning (*see* pp 6, 7). There were the participants returning from courses who reported back to their colleagues (*see* p 9), the podiatrist who taught the doctor and nurse how to examine the foot (*see* p 9), the GP who went away to read up the answer to the practice nurse's question (*see* p 30) and another who made time to explain to the secretary-receptionist how the printer worked (*see* p 51) – interprofessional learning at its most basic, but also its best.

Work-located interprofessional learning is often equated with teambuild-ing, although that term found few friends when advice from opinion leaders was canvassed.[12] Preoccupations with 'team' as a concept could, said some, divert attention from the job in hand. Many preferred task-centred approaches rather than teambuilding exercises, thought by some inadvertently to alienate members from each other. Task-centred learning set aside differences to deliver outcomes, differences that only needed to be addressed if and when they impeded progress, at which point lessons might be learned with wider applica-tion. Team development more aptly describes the learning in action that has characterised work based interprofessional learning since primary care centres first began to be established in the 1960s.

Horder recalls how it was unusual in the 1950s in his London practice for GPs to meet or speak with district nurses, health visitors or social workers deal-ing with the same patient.[13] Contact between doctor and nurse often took the form of notes left for each other on the mantelpiece at the patient's home!

Communications began to improve, said Horder, when nurses, and health visitors (and occasionally social workers) were attached to particular practices and, more firmly, when they began to work under the same roof. But the most important change came when they started to meet regularly to discuss organisational problems and shared responsibility for patients.

Effective teamwork, Horder found, depended, first, upon communication and, second, upon continuity, before members were willing to reveal themselves without fear of criticism or contempt. An important test of team cohesion was the degree to which ignorance, mistakes and failures could be revealed and discussed.

The immediate objective for a discussion might be to agree the best solution to a clinical problem, but the longer-term benefit lay in enabling team members to develop their confidence and thinking. The team had two overall purposes: to provide the best possible service to the practice population and to create a place of work in which everyone was learning and developing.

A monthly cycle of meetings was introduced into a four-doctor semi-rural practice in Northumberland in order to strengthen teamwork and to cope with the demands of new contracts, which necessitated change at a frightening pace. Each meeting lasted for an hour over Friday lunchtime.

Week one was a staff meeting, week two a primary healthcare team business meeting, week three an interprofessional educational meeting and week four a doctors' meeting.

Two district nurses, one practice nurse, four GPs, one trainee GP, two health visitors and a community midwife participated in the educational meetings.

The aims were:

- to improve knowledge, skills and attitudes
- to improve working together through learning together
- to improve the way that the practice operated
- to increase job satisfaction.

Participants divided into groups of three during the first meeting to define their educational needs and to discuss appropriate learning methods. A format of small-group work, presentations and guest speakers was agreed. Responsibility for organising sessions was delegated to individuals or pairs.

The first series of meetings during 1991–2 consisted of a varied diet of topics covering clinical, organisational and personal aspects of the team's work.

Improving asthma care was singled out as an important clinical objective. The practice nurse and a GP led the session based upon an audit of asthma care and informed by relevant articles distributed in advance for preliminary reading. Emerging themes were presented, deemed to characterise good asthma care. Participants then split into small groups to list those tasks to be undertaken each year with an asthmatic patient to provide a good standard of care. The session ended by compiling a checklist to be used by all staff in future contacts with asthmatic patients and agreeing to review progress at a future meeting.

Anonymous evaluation followed each session. Comments and ratings were collated and fed back to session leaders and speakers. Participants were also asked to complete a questionnaire at the end of the first programme. Findings suggested 'a reasonably good level of satisfaction'. Two sessions stood out, one on stress management (which scored highly for enjoyment!), the other on the management of a terminally ill patient thought to have confirmed the value of the team approach. Some sessions were, however, thought to be over-ambitious, throwing up more issues than could be resolved there and then, and resulting in frustration.[14]

I chose the above example in the expectation that it would provide a familiar starting point from which to explore more sophisticated approaches to work-located learning.

The Monkfield Medical Practice was established in the year 2000 on a green-field site near Cambridge. The 'lead partner' wanted the team to include a range of professional expertise to provide broadly based healthcare services. It comprised two doctors, two nurse practitioners, a child/family nurse, a clinical pharmacist, a Well Family Service co-ordinator, a service development manager, a research and learning officer, a patient participation co-ordinator, an information technology co-ordinator and administrative staff.

Team members were attracted by the opportunity to develop new approaches to practice, but some experienced periods of self-doubt as they questioned their capacity to address the roles that they had assumed. Attempts were made to understand the problems in one-to-one discussions in a supportive no-blame culture. Many of the relevant training opportunities identified related to new roles, notably that of nurse practitioner.

Members were encouraged to maintain strong and continuing links with their 'base' professions. External mentors were found from each profession and their role integrated into internal professional development and appraisal mechanisms.

Potential conflicts were addressed arising from allegiances and accountability outside the team by canvassing the views of 'partner employers' to understand better their expectations, while a 360-degree reflective development process encompassed some of the appraisal requirements operated by external partners within the one developed for the practice. This enabled team members to review the entirety of their contribution rather than its dismembered parts.

Problems rarely presented themselves clearly. Undercurrents of concern and discomfort were identified which called for teamworking towards a clearer understanding as members found a safe channel through hidden hazards in uncharted waters.[15]

Few examples could capture better how a primary care centre can become a learning organisation, sensitive and responsive to the moods and feelings of its workers, identifying problems, encouraging reflection without threatening, translating working problems into learning needs, mobilising internal and external training resources, respecting and reinforcing the professional identity of each worker, and reconciling individual and organisational agendas.

More sophisticated approaches to work-located learning owe much to developments following the recommendation in a report from the Chief Medical Officer for England for practice professional development planning (PPDP).[16]

A feasibility study in Wales sought to integrate professional and practice development planning to resolve the mismatch between changing clinical practice and attendance at passive educational events. A team of facilitators worked with 12 general practices, of varying size, degrees of organisational development and sophistication, over 12 months, applying the PPDP change process.

The objectives were the same in each case:

- to secure the production of a practice development plan
- to develop skills in building consensus and shared objectives
- to recognise the value of the network contribution to problem solving and learning
- to achieve at least one organisational improvement
- to promote great organisational integration
- to establish a systematic 'plan–do–review' approach to organisational development.

Each practice had five facilitated 'time out' sessions lasting half a day. The first was devoted to the identification of specific organisational needs employing collaborative enquiry[17,18] designed to ensure that everyone contributed, selecting one priority by the end. During the second session the chosen priority was analysed using a predetermined protocol. Practices identified the criteria against which their performance would be judged and to provide a focus for subsequent reflection. Participants were then asked to document the necessary personal developments required to enable the practice to deliver its chosen objective. Progress was reviewed by means of iterative experiential and reflective cycles, identifying further work to be done. Finally, the transferability of the learning process to other developments was considered.

Reviewing their role, the facilitators distinguished between initiating, sustaining and process design phases.[19]

During the initiating phase, they found that many of the GPs were uncomfortable in making time to participate, which they regarded as a drain on already limited time for patient care. PPDP had to be made relevant to patient care. Time required needed to be 'ring fenced' to engage productively in PPDP.

During the sustaining phase, suppressed internal conflicts surfaced, as did struggles to retain power and outright refusal to co-operate. Some GPs 'took the risk' of inviting employed and attached staff to participate, only to feel exposed or threatened. Winning consensus proved more difficult, but outcomes proved more beneficial in promoting teamwork and cohesion. Moreover, involving the wider team added energy and momentum to the PPDP process. Many individuals, particularly in non-clinical roles, were found to have a wealth of experience to contribute, but lacked the confidence without encouragement.

Projects that established a core group faced difficulty in communicating the rationale and process for the chosen development to the 'grass-roots' and across disciplinary boundaries.

During the process design phase, questions of authority and control again proved to be problematic, especially where GPs played an autocratic role and/ or projects involved cross-boundary and inter-agency working. The facilitators observed that GPs operate, often informally and implicitly, an internal governance framework as partners and owners of the business. Project subgroups that conflicted with this governance framework risked challenge, a risk that increased with the growing confidence, capability and independence of the project teams. The hardest thing of all was to convince primary care organisations that collaboration was worth the effort. Practices did not instinctively value an organic, self-directed, iterative process of learning.

General practice, the facilitators concluded, was ridden with conflict between the values of individual practitioners and of the organisation, a conflict held in creative tension whose energy PPDP could release.[20–22]

Work-located learning may be self-sufficient and self-contained, but the last two examples break free from that narrow view, calling as they did upon external facilitators and mentors, and, in Monkfield, releasing workers to attend external courses. Such work-related learning may well be uni-professional to reinforce and update profession-specific knowledge and skills. Work-related interprofessional learning is, however, more relevant in this chapter.

Work-related learning

The classic role for work-related interprofessional learning is to create time and space to reflect upon practice, based upon the assumption that this is lacking in the workplace. Arguably, the more successful practices become in building in opportunities for reflective learning, the less need they have to release workers to attend work-related courses. That, however, overlooks the qualitative difference between the two learning environments.

Learning at work is essentially tied to the here and now demands of practice between immediate colleagues. Objectives are typically short-term and task-specific.

Learning away from the job offers the chance to stand back, to see the wood from the trees, to compare approaches to similar problems in different agencies, to think the unthinkable without fear of reproach, on neutral ground. It can also take the longer-term view, looking beyond needs and expectations of the present post, work setting or agency.

Just as I took a simple example to introduce work-located learning, so the following example does the same for work-related learning.

> The Marylebone Centre Trust invited a range of workers from primary health and community care to one of two workshops held in the early 1990s. There they were encouraged to present examples of current work which involved a high degree of collaboration across professional and agency boundaries, identifying what helped and hindered collaboration, to explore implications for interprofessional education and training.
>
> The workshops followed an action and reflection cycle. Action took the form of presentations by participants on topics ranging from open referral in mental health to meeting the needs of long-term housebound people, and from working with carers to multidisciplinary approaches to health promotion. Reflection took the form of small-group discussion, feedback from the observer and reports back from sub-groups.
>
> Among the issues discussed were: the impact of policy and organisational change on professional roles; professional differences as difficulty and opportunity; differences in language, culture and values; communication and negotiation between professions; and leadership in collaborative projects.[23,24]

Workshops such as this encourage participants to call upon practice and, hopefully, prepare them when they return to their places of work to engage in change, armed with enhanced understanding, skills and motivation – 'hopefully' because there can be no guarantee that participants will be so motivated, nor that the agency will be receptive.

> A groundbreaking series of workshops convened by the Health Education Authority (HEA) sought to overcome these weaknesses. Joint applications were invited from colleagues in primary care from different professions. Each group committed itself from the outset to devise a strategy for change to be developed during the workshop and to be implemented subsequently, so far as practicable, in the knowledge that colleagues had promised support in advance.
>
> Eighteen workshops were mounted as a rolling programme during the 1980s to generate health promotion in primary care throughout England.

At least three participants came from the same primary care team, including GPs, nurses, health visitors, practice managers, administrators and secretaries. Each workshop lasted two days, each team selecting its own topic for health promotion in its practice. Applying principles of adult learning, the workshops valued and utilised the knowledge and skills that the participants brought with them. Learning was facilitative, participative, collaborative, reflective and exploratory, employing problem solving to develop teamwork.

Facilitators offered each group help in establishing its baselines, locating target audiences, identifying inhibiting and enabling factors, and devising means of evaluation before returning home to implement its plans.[25]

Nine more workshops followed for local organising teams (LOTs) charged with responsibility for multiplying the benefits of the learning approach. Projects generated covered a wide spectrum, reflecting contemporary pre-occupations in primary care – management systems, computerisation, audit and evaluation, patient education and the needs of minority ethnic groups as well as health promotion and coronary heart disease which had featured strongly in the HEA programme.[26]

The HEA strategy achieved more than any other initiative in implanting a learning culture throughout primary care nationwide, generating a cohort of some 50 freelance facilitators by the late 1980s upon whom practices continued to call. Much of their work in the early years took the form of consultancy and training, especially for practice nurses, helping them to overcome their isolation and acquire knowledge and skills to develop their role.[27]

Many of these freelancers joined the National Facilitators Development Project at the HEA primary healthcare unit in Oxford,[28,29] or formed collectives such as LOTUS based in Sheffield. This group comprised ten facilitators with a co-ordinator. They worked in pairs from different professions to offer up to six two-hour workshops to primary healthcare teams. Each team selected its own learning topic and reflective learning plan. Topics chosen ranged from communication skills to dealing with violent patients and from staff mentoring to change management.[30]

Integrating work-located and work-related learning

Developments in the south west of England are remarkable for the manner in which they integrate work-located and work-related learning, based upon partnership between practice agencies and universities driven by continuous quality improvement methods (CQI) introduced from the United States.

Widespread adoption of CQI in healthcare in the USA owes much to the lead given by the Interdisciplinary Professions Education Collaborative (IPEC) launched by the Institute for Health Improvement (IHI) during the 1990s with federal government support.[31] It followed the collapse of the healthcare reforms proposed by the Clinton administration, providing an alternative springboard for change from the grass-roots.

The NHS South West sent delegates to IPEC conferences in the USA. Close working relationships were forged as a result and linked initiatives launched across the Atlantic as reported in a special issue of the *Journal of Interprofessional Care*.[32]

The NHS Regional Office had become increasingly concerned about poor recruitment to many of the supposedly interprofessional continuing education courses that it funded in universities. Disappointing recruitment often failed to attract the intended professional mix, some courses being limited to different branches of nursing.[33,34]

Searching for an alternative strategy, and impressed by early initiatives in CQI in the region, the Regional Office decided to concentrate available funds on a number of sustainable and systematic developments clustered around three centres, each based upon a partnership between a university and health and social care agencies. The aim was to introduce new models to effect improvements in interprofessional learning, practice and patient care by establishing local improvement teams (LITs), which would apply CQI. The three centres operated as a collaborative, exchanging experience, working together to resolve problems and accounting to the same board.[35]

Three universities – Bournemouth, Plymouth and the West of England – took part in the three-year project funded by the NHS Executive South West, forming LITs, each including a minimum of three professions.

Twelve teachers from Bournemouth University, drawn from different disciplines, worked with health and social care agencies in three locations. In Andover, the focus was upon improving support for parents of young children, in Dorchester upon improving care for acutely ill elderly people in hospital and in Salisbury upon improving community mental health care. All comprised action learning sets, employed CQI and actively involved service users.

Health studies, social and medical schools at the University of Plymouth worked through three committees to improve participation by users in services for people with severe and enduring mental health problems and to develop modules to incorporate into undergraduate and postgraduate courses.

The University of the West of England worked with experienced practitioners from agencies in Avon, Somerset and Wiltshire to establish action learning sets to make care for people with cancer more sensitive and more responsive by understanding the lived experience of service users who took part and employing a CQI cycle.

The projects taught that interprofessional learning was not about fudging boundaries or creating generic workers, but developing professionals who were confident in their core skills and expertise, aware of and having confidence in the skills and expertise of other professions, and able to conduct their practice in a non-hierarchical and collegiate way with other team members.[35,36]

These are just some of the CQI projects in the region. Another has been written up more fully.

Five general practices joined forces with support from Bournemouth University to establish the Dorset Seedcorn Project. Groups were drawn from each practice, comprising at least one GP principal, one nurse and one administrator, with others as appropriate. Each designed and implemented an agreed change in services to patients employing an accelerated model for quality improvement, helped by a facilitator from the university, and in the expectation that the experience would lead to more effective teamwork. Help from colleagues was co-opted to effect implementation.

The following 'topics' were chosen for improvement:

- handling patients' telephone enquiries on clinical matters
- improving a service for acutely ill under-fives
- addressing the needs of frequent attenders
- improving care for elderly residents in a social services home
- improving services for adolescents in a social service assessment centre.

Larger teams were then convened, calling upon members from inside and outside the practices. Hopes, expectations and anxieties were exchanged, ground rules formulated and points identified where change might have greatest benefit. Measures were then agreed to gauge progress, review the process and identify next steps.

Follow-up eight months later found that all plans had been implemented and changes integrated into everyday work. Practices reported benefits in clinical management strategy, collaborative practice and staff satisfaction.

Participants were positive about using a similar process to effect change in the future and some practices had already done so. Patients valued improvements in services, while staff of the two social services establishments reported better relations with practices, resulting in better services for their residents.[37]

Some readers may question whether these developments count as work-located learning. Others may see them as a quantum leap, redefining and reversing the traditional relationship between learning and practice. That view is widely held in the south west and by its American partners, a view that is winning friends as the methodology is adopted elsewhere.

One more development in the south west merits mention, namely the way in which the work-located CQI projects contribute to pre-registration studies. Many take students on placement, introducing them to quality improvement as an essential part of their professional competence,[36,38] while the teachers assigned to the projects introduce CQI into their pre-registration college teaching. The more teachers engage in work-located learning, the more informed they become about the demands of contemporary practice and the better prepared they are to modify pre-registration studies accordingly.

References

1 CAIPE (1997) Interprofessional education – a definition. *CAIPE Bulletin.* **13**: 19.

2 Shakespeare H, Tucker W and Northover J (1989) *Report of a National Survey on Interprofessional Education in Primary Care.* CAIPE, London.

3 Barr H and Waterton S (1996) *Interprofessional Education in Health and Social Care in the United Kingdom: report of a CAIPE survey.* CAIPE, London.

4 Barr H (2002) *Interprofessional Education Today, Yesterday and Tomorrow.* LTSN Centre for Health Sciences and Practice, London.

5 Hewstone M and Brown RJ (1986) Contact is not enough: an intergroup perspective on the 'contact hypothesis'. In: M Hewstone and RJ Brown (eds) *Contact and Conflict in Intergroup Encounter.* Blackwell, Oxford.

6 Tajfel H (1981) *Human Groups and Social Categories.* Cambridge University Press, Cambridge.

7 Carpenter J (1995) Interprofessional education for medical and nursing students: evaluation of a programme. *Medical Education.* **29**: 265–72.

8 Carpenter J (1995) Doctors and nurses: stereotypes and stereotype change in interprofessional education. *J Interprofessional Care.* **9**: 151–62.

9 Carpenter J and Hewstone M (1996) Shared learning for doctors and social workers. *Br J Social Work.* **26**: 239–57.

10 McMichael P, Irvine R and Gilloran A (1984) *Pathways to the Professions: Research Report.* Moray House College of Education, Edinburgh.

11 Barnes D, Carpenter J and Dickinson C (2000) Interprofessional education for community mental health: attitudes to community care and professional stereotypes. *Social Work Education.* **19**: 565–83.

12 Barr H (1994) *Perspectives on Shared Learning.* CAIPE, London.

13 Horder J (2000) Leadership in a multiprofessional context. *Medical Education.* **34(3)**: 203–5.

14 Cunningham W (1995) Interdisciplinary practice educational meetings – continuing education for the working primary health care team. *Education for General Practice.* 6: 41–8.

15 Bateman H, Bailey P and McLellan H (forthcoming) Of rocks and safe channels: learning to navigate as an interprofessional team. *J Interprofessional Care.*

16 Department of Health (1998) *A Review of Continuing Professional Development in Practice: a report of the Chief Medical Officer.* HMSO, London.

17 Reason P (1986) Innovative research techniques. *Complementary Medical Research.* 1: 23–39.

18 Reason P (1999) Integrating education and reflection through co-operative inquiry. *Management Learning.* 30: 207–26.

19 Senge P, Kleiner A, Roberts C et al. (1999) *The Dance of Change; the challenge of sustaining momentum in learning organisations.* Routledge, London.

20 Carlisle S, Elwyn G and Smail S (2000) Personal practice development plans in primary care in Wales. *J Interprofessional Care.* 14: 39–48.

21 Burtonwood AM, Hocking PJ and Elwyn G (2001) Joining them up: the challenges of organisational change in the professional politic of general practice. *J Interprofessional Care.* 15: 383–93.

22 Elwyn G, Hocking P, Burtonwood A et al. (forthcoming) Learning to plan? A critical fiction about the facilitation of professional and practice development plans in primary care. *J Interprofessional Care.*

23 Spratley J and Pietroni M (1994) *Creative Learning: interprofessional learning priorities in primary health and community care.* Marylebone Centre Trust, London.

24 Barr H and Shaw I (1995) *Shared Learning: selected examples from the literature.* CAIPE, London.

25 Spratley J (1990) *Disease Prevention and Health Promotion in Primary Health.* Health Education Authority, London.

26 Spratley J (1990) *Joint Planning for the Development and Management of Disease Prevention and Health Promotion Strategies in Primary Health Care.* Health Education Authority, London.

27 Astrop P (1988) What the facilitator can do for the practice nurse. *Practice Nurse.* May: 13–17.

28 Fullard E, Fowler G and Gray M (1984) Facilitating prevention in primary care. *BMJ.* 289: 1585–7.

29 Fullard, E, Fowler G and Grey M (1987) Promoting prevention in primary care: controlled trial of low technology, low cost approach. *BMJ.* 294: 1080–2.

30 Pirie Z and Basford L (1998) LOTUS delivering CPD to teams. *CAIPE Bulletin.* 15: 16–17.

31 Schmitt MH (2000) Continuous quality improvement in health professions education. *J Interprofessional Care.* 14(2): 109–10.

32 Wilcock PM and Headrick LA (2000) Interprofessional learning for the improvement of health care: why bother? *J Interprofessional Care.* 14: 111–17.

33 Tope R (1999) *The Impact of Inter-professional Education Projects in the South West Region: a critical analysis.* NHS South West, Bristol.

34 Tope R (2001) *Inter-professional Education in the South West Region 1999–2000.* NHS South West, Bristol.

35 NHS South West (2001) *Interprofessional Education.* NHS South West, Bristol.

36 Annandale S, McCann S, Nattrass H *et al.* (2000) Achieving health improvement through interprofessional learning in south west England. *J Interprofessional Care.* **14**: 161–74.

37 Campion-Smith C and Wilcock PM (2000) Interprofessional learning and continuous quality improvement in primary care: the Dorset Seedcorn Project. *CAIPE Bulletin.* **18**: 11–12.

38 Wilcock P and Lewis A (2002) Putting improvement at the heart of health care. *BMJ.* **325**: 670–1.

Acknowledgement

I am indebted to Dr John Horder for his critique of this chapter in draft and for suggesting additional sources.

CHAPTER 7

Learning from patients

Penny Morris and Penny Trafford

Where Osler could treat patients as passive consumers of care which doctors devised and nurses implemented, but patients unquestioningly endured, we must accept patients as colleagues in a jointly designed and performed production, in which they will nearly always have to do most of the work. (Julian Tudor Hart)

Preparing the ground

The authors of this chapter write as community based practitioners and educationalists. Penny Morris works on improving communication between health professionals and patients: this work is rooted in her experience in community development in Salford and Chicago; Penny Trafford is a GP principal in North London, involved in practice based learning and development. We have both worked with initiatives to involve patients and the general public directly in attempts to help health professionals learn and change. Most of the examples and vignettes which illustrate these themes in the chapter come from this work. We also examine what makes for successful learning from patients in WBL. We examine this in the context of the developing culture of primary care and changing relationships between health professionals and their patients.

We use the word 'patients' as a generic term for the public to whom health professionals relate. We concentrate on the different roles that patients can play in helping professionals learn in the new world of primary healthcare. We also use the word 'healing' in this chapter. By and large, we use healing to describe the capacity of patients to take charge of and make sense of their own illnesses and to participate in the process of recovery.

NHS policy makers have exhorted health planners and providers to involve patients and the public in all aspects of healthcare.[1] A growing body of work from policy academics identifies *'a need to change the culture, attitudes and behaviour of those providing the service'*.[2]

There is a small but expanding literature about learning from patients and how such learning can contribute to these changes. This is our perspective. We use a community development approach that aims to empower not only patients, but also the practitioners. Much of the commentary on the professional/patient relationship is critical of professionals. We take a different view, as we think that if one starts from a critical viewpoint, then it is difficult to make progress. Rather, we like to draw on the strengths of the health teams with which we work. Almost always, they already possess the capacity to listen, empathise and problem solve.

There is, however, some resistance to listening to patients in such a way that patients' ideas and concerns are fully recognised and acknowledged. Our experience has shown us that ways of learning are required which enable professionals first to find their own voice to express their ideas and concerns about this whole prospect of developing partnerships with patients.

In addition, we think that learning from patients is more than just allocating space to the patient's story. Listening means that the patient's story becomes a way for the professional to learn – to learn about an illness, human psychology, an individual's experiences of life, or better methods of treatment. In this way, listening to patients contributes to the development of the professional. The patient, by the same token, feels better understood, better accepted and, in short, becomes empowered by the experience and can experience healing. This is in line with other initiatives supported by both government and patient groups.[3]

Professionals already learn from their daily encounters with patients: it is 'inescapable', as described in the Introduction. Professionals also learn from their own experiences of patient-hood. These ways of learning are well documented in contexts where professionals' stories are told – for example, in the Personal View section of the *British Medical Journal*.

But many professionals have not learned to trust their own experience. They are overly influenced by a clinical education that emphasises the idea of the 'right answer' at the expense of considering the complexities of human responses to ill health.[4] Such past learning experiences hinder some aspects of the personal and professional development of health professionals.

As discussed in Chapter 3 in this book, Linden West describes this process for doctors as the 'profound split between personhood and medical practice'.[5] Such a split can lead to a fundamental disregard of what patients as people say, in favour of some other interpretation or expertise. This disregard has implications for every aspect of healthcare. When the voice of the person within the patient is silenced in the culture of primary care, it means avoiding the patient perspective in clinical encounters, resisting patients' suggestions for practice improvement and ignoring patients' views in policy and planning.

Learning together as a primary healthcare team is a relatively new concept to many healthcare professionals. Most practices are still developing patient participation within their organisation. The idea that patients could be actively involved in WBL is revolutionary for many. For some professionals the notion of working in partnership with patients is threatening and unwanted.[6] Others have found that having a more equal relationship with patients makes their work more productive and rewarding.[7]

The evidence base for sharing information and decision making with patients in clinical consultations is growing.[8] It seems, however, that the majority of younger professionals still do not involve patients in making decisions nor check that they have understood information that has been given, despite the teaching of patient-centred care in vocational training and nursing training.[9]

This may be because the idea of involving patients fully in clinical encounters, working with their perspective to explore and solve problems, is interpreted as adding to professionals' burden of care, rather than being a matter of sharing responsibility and easing the burden for professionals and patients.[10] 'Blocking behaviour' is used by professionals as a defence against this 'burden'.[4,11]

We argue that involving patients as active partners in learning organisations can help change this construct. Work based, interprofessional learning with an empowered patient voice could help shape the new delivery of primary healthcare to the benefit of all.

We will describe examples of patient involvement at different levels of learning encounter. We have found, echoing others' experience, that significant learning from patients can take place in:

- face-to-face clinical encounters and the reviewing of these
- practice development
- wider primary care development.

Thus patients, the focus of health professionals' work, are potential partners of health professionals in that very work. As partners they can work together to set common goals. A key task for educationalists is to nurture the mutual respect required for patients and professionals to work together.

Research has suggested that there are core principles for good practice to ensure this. These principles include the following.

- Preparing patients and professionals for partnership: this means giving both parties a voice to express their creative ideas and difficult feelings.
- Involving patients near the beginning of any learning or development exercise, to help set the agenda.
- Giving opportunities to reflect on personal practice and experiment with new ways of seeing and behaving.
- Establishing clear structures to encourage a feeling of safety and openness to change.
- Encouraging professionals and patients in WBL to support each other to build on their strengths. This parallels and reinforces an empowerment model for individual patients.

- Making sure that agreed outcomes from shared learning and development are jointly evaluated and followed up.

The rest of this chapter outlines some of the differing roles patients can play in healthcare, and their changing relationships with primary care professionals. It then discusses ways of preparing professionals and patients for partnership. We explore how patients can help professionals to learn from face-to-face clinical encounters. We also explore how patients can facilitate practice development and wider primary care development. We describe work we have undertaken and relate it to the research of others. Finally, we point out how patients can contribute not only to the performance of professionals but also to their well-being.

Different roles, changing relationships

The NHS workforce has experienced dramatic and accelerating attempts at change in the last few years promoted by government.[12] This is in the context of new guidelines being set by government for the delivery of national healthcare targets, with the subsequent re-evaluation of the nature and role of health professionals themselves. Government strategy has been shaped partly by fiscal pressures to contain costs and yet respond to escalating patient expectations of treatment. It has also been shaped by anxieties about the misuse of power by professionals.[13] Such anxiety has developed in parallel with the growing availability of knowledge about health and medicine through the Internet and other media with which patients increasingly arm themselves before consultations.

Other social changes have encouraged different thinking about the patient's part in care. In current models of 'autonomous'[14] and 'resourceful'[15] patients, the professional is likened to a sensitive mechanic, offering appropriate services to patients who have been empowered with resources to take more charge of their own health and care.

These paradigms for patient/professional relationships have developed out of movements for change inside the NHS since the 1960s and 1970s.

Professional power over health decision making began to be actively challenged by lobbies such as the feminist health and mental health movements. With the support of campaigning health professionals, changes in healthcare have resulted, such as the less medicalised delivery of care in childbirth and the growth of the social psychiatry model within therapeutic communities, together with the development of patient participation groups attached to general practice surgeries. In 1974, Community Health Councils were established to provide local people with a voice in healthcare. Many of the leading and influential advocates for change in 21st-century healthcare have their roots in these alternative social programmes.

By the 1980s and 1990s there were further pressures for change from growing consumerist awareness and the movement of patient self-help groups around specific illnesses. The Patient's Charter was issued calling for an increased use of patient evaluations of services. Later, these efforts to improve matters for individual patients were complemented by more government-led community approaches to developing partnership with patients. These included focus groups, citizen juries and local health panels. At the same time, voluntary groups and professionals collaborated in projects to improve health for communities.[16]

Following the launch of *The New NHS* in 1997, health providers are now required to demonstrate their attempts at patient and public involvement from board level downwards.[1] These initiatives may, however, be token in nature, given the growing influence of consumerism and competition in the health service.[17]

This history means that the daily working reality of primary care professionals now includes dealing with a wide and evolving range of patient perceptions and behaviours, while the boundaries of their own professional roles are shifting.

Framing the patient role

There are many ways of framing the patient role. One helpful way is to consider what is possible for patients and the public as *clients, consumers* or *citizens* in healthcare.[18] *Clients* traditionally play no role in evaluating the solutions to their problems, let alone deciding on the solution or even defining the problem. *Consumers* can evaluate solutions but the availability of choices is limited by the provider. *Citizens* in healthcare, on the other hand, join in to set the agenda, define the problem and evaluate the solution.

In the present experimental world of primary healthcare we, like others, have found that regarding patients as citizens is helpful to successful learning from patients.[19] This means acknowledging and developing patients' capacities in order to enable them to contribute at every level of encounter, including face to face.

We mentioned earlier how patients can go unheard during primary care encounters. Practitioners working from a 'narrative base' take care to elicit and help develop patients' stories in the context of their family and community. John Launer[20] describes how:

> *Empowerment of the patient is clearly at the heart of the narrative approach. Every technique is aimed at helping the patient to lead the narrative, and to share in the choices and dilemmas that have to be addressed. Empowerment is not just about sharing the final decision about what to do. It is about looking for opportunities at every moment to hand over power. Nowhere is this more important than in the minute-to-minute conduct of the consultation itself.*

The 'citizen' concept of the patient is also consistent with the model of consultations as 'meetings between experts' where sharing understanding is the key task.[21] Such a model is used in the current curricula for communication skills teaching in UK medical schools.

One government initiative which directly supports learning from patients as experts is the paper *The Expert Patient*.[3] This builds on the strengths of patient self-help groups and is directed at preparing those with chronic illness to become enablers of other patients, sharing ideas for self-care. We describe later how 'expert patients' also help professionals to learn.

Drawing on already existing skills

Most health professionals have developed considerable skills in helping patients sort out complex areas of health and illness, even if they frequently decline to use such skills. When practitioners, working in groups, undertake a reflective and facilitated study of difficult consultations, we have found that they often make an important connection.[7] They discover that there is a parallel between how they help each other to untangle problems in a learning group of this kind and the way that they, as individual practitioners, can work with patients to untangle a problem. For individual practitioners such workshops can lead to a significant development experience and have been described as leading to a change of ideas and a transformation of practice.[22] Professionals learn to use their already existing skills to develop their patients' resources. They use essentially educational approaches with their patients, approaches that support learning for change.

Preparing to learn from patients

The practice team

The principle of drawing on already existing skills also applies to helping professionals learn from patients as a group. For example, recently, the NHS Executive, London Region, commissioned a working party to create a programme that would enable practitioners in primary care to embrace patient/public participation.[6] The programme has now been rolled out to primary care trusts (PCTs). The working party concluded that the programme would start from the perspective that practice teams need to be prepared for learning from and sharing decision making with patients about the services they provide. This is because professional, clinical and managerial staff may be unprepared, unaware and, at times, hostile to public participation. Attempts to involve the 'public' on professional and managerial committees often end in frustration on both sides. Previous work sought to address this by training the lay participants.[23]

The aim of this programme is to help primary healthcare professionals to examine their attitudes to patient participation and critically to appraise the culture within the practice team. Two people from each practice in a PCT attend seven sessions with work in between sessions. The group discusses the reasons for partnership, providing information for patients, the patient's journey, feedback from patients and working with community groups.

The goal is to give practice staff the confidence to undertake change and to see the benefits to them of a less hierarchical, more patient-focused organisation.

Those who developed the programme identify the following stages to its success.

- First, it is important to give professionals the opportunity to explore anxieties about involving patients. The group often feels threatened and worried about being overwhelmed by patients' demands. The practice team can see itself joined against a common enemy that might be the patients, the system or the government imposing this agenda. These feelings need to be expressed and understood.
- Second, it is useful to emphasise building on what practices do already. This can be facilitated by:

    - encouraging positive reflection on the details of daily practice for the team
    - talking about enlarging the area of overlap between patients' needs and those of the practice
    - sharing good ideas.

The aim is to help professionals move towards a constructive dialogue with patients about the development of their services. The process increases reflection by the team and enables learning from patients by the primary care organisation.

This patient input can result in practice development. For example, one practice team, which had been involved in the experience outlined earlier, decided to discuss the issue of the changing role of the health visitor. A steering committee was formed involving members of the primary healthcare team and patients. The steering committee was empowered to suggest and implement some changes and to design the future of the baby clinics in response to feedback. The changing role of health visitors in the new NHS had been recognised among the practice team. The health visitor brought the following problems to the attention of a practice meeting:

- the recent discontinuation of routine monitoring of families at home
- the probable imminent disappearance of routine child surveillance
- the need for a review of baby clinics from the patient's perspective – do they meet the needs of children and parents in their present form?

At present the practice is developing a proposal to address these issues.

Undergraduate education and vocational training

Lack of appropriate training in how to work in partnership with patients still prevents the appropriate use of patients' expertise and wisdom.[24]

Student and trainee health professionals, like practising professionals, cannot help but learn from their encounters with patients. But traditionally patients have been regarded as passive and have usually acted simply as a vehicle or medium through which the clinical teacher teaches. This means that the potential for patients' contribution during early education and training and later work based learning has been missed. The notion that they can give another, equally valuable, perspective to learning has grown as the traditional role of the patient has developed.[25] The recognition of the importance of the patients' expertise in their experience of illness has not only changed teaching about clinical consultations, it has also resulted in the idea of the expert patient as a more responsible partner in care and as an independent teacher.

For example, on a GP vocational training scheme, a number of patients were present. Each patient taught a group of GP registrars about his or her experience of a chronic illness. RS has rheumatoid arthritis. She demonstrated the clinical signs in her hands: muscle wasting, deformity of joints, swan neck in her index finger and ulnar deviation of all her fingers, and explained how this affects the activities of daily living. She talked about the treatment given and the side effects. There was discussion around the impact of her illness on her lifestyle and relationships, and she answered the doctors' questions.

A fuller understanding of patients' and communities' roles in healing is one key to this change. We described earlier a notion of the citizenship of patients in healthcare, where people's capacities for solving problems are respected and tended. Wykurz argues that if patients are regarded as equal citizens in educating professionals, this shift in status will reflect the shift in attitudes of those leading the teaching.[26] The capacities of patients and communities will be recognised, as well as their problems.

Increasingly, students visit patients, patient groups and community organisations, in people's homes and community venues. There they can learn to appreciate patients' own resources for healing, which can complement the expertise of the professional. This helps to unlock the burdensome notion that professionals are the only source of help.[10]

Patients as teachers

Through interaction between students and patients on patients' own ground rather than in hospital beds, the role of patients as active teachers has grown.

For example, during one project, Patients as Partners, patients with chronic illnesses were visited several times by medical students. Their patient partners helped them set learning objectives and also assessed them.[26] In nursing education, the involvement of patients as teachers has been established as a priority.[27] There have been various schemes which have explored how educational institutions could best support nurses in learning from patients.[28]

With its history of influencing psychiatric practice, user involvement in the field of mental health is particularly well developed. This extends to service provision in primary care (by users), as well as service planning and evaluation. Educational initiatives involving users in this field are more likely to be user-led.[29]

One of the largest groups of lay people directly involved in health professional education is the growing body of 'simulated patients'. These are people from the local community, sometimes actors, who are recruited and trained by universities and vocational training schemes to role-play as patients in practice consultations. The membership examination for general practice includes a simulated GP surgery option where the simulated patients contribute to the assessment of candidates.

Those involved in these developments recognise that there should be wider representation of their local communities in such teaching. It will be important for educationalists to establish effective partnerships with local people. This has been done successfully; for example, in 1978, a community drama group based in Manchester (North West Spanner) started to help the university's Department of General Practice with a new project. Members of the group role-played patients so that medical students could practise consultations. Led by David Metcalfe, the department had a history of investigating how doctors listen to patients and were committed to engaging with their community.[30] Collaboration between the GP teachers and the drama group was fruitful, based on mutual respect. It became clear that the drama group members were bringing to the teaching their own experience of working with groups in the community. They offered a lay perspective to role development and feedback, and became teachers in their own right, not merely audiovisual aids. They felt that they were always treated as equal colleagues. They have continued to extend this work nationwide.[31]

Here are some points summarising what is needed to help patients and the public teach effectively.

- Prepare the ground: involve patients near the beginning of any learning exercise, to help set the teaching agenda and identify the resources needed to deliver it.
- Ensure they have the information and resources they need to help students learn.
- Jointly evaluate the learning.

Changing clinical encounters between patients and professionals

Part of the difficulty lies in doctors' attitudes and reluctance to relinquish power or to reveal the true level of uncertainty that often exists in clinical decision making.[32]

One of the cornerstones of effective WBL is the acknowledgement of uncertainty. It is on this aspect of the work that this section focuses. Uncertainty increases as information about the latest discoveries in healthcare proliferates for professionals and their patients. We have described how doctors often fail to acknowledge patients' own expertise in their condition and their knowledge about their own needs. Doctors and nurses may also find it hard to adjust to those who are well informed about clinical aspects of care, as they can find them threatening. For the professional not to know the answer to clinical queries is felt as shaming. In Chapter 1 in this book, the professional 'bluff' as self-defence is described: when a nurse was questioned by a relative about the management of prostate cancer, the nurse found a way to avoid revealing that she did not know the answer.

Vignette 7.1
One GP has found in her own practice that she can put the effort she used to spend during consultations on avoiding revelation of her uncertainty into exploring what the patient is thinking.

She had treated a young man with dyspepsia, who was *Helicobacter* positive on serum analysis, with triple therapy. Two weeks later she received a message to phone him.

Doctor: *How can I help?*
Patient: *When do I have my breath test?*
Doctor: *Sorry?* (Her thoughts were: is this a doctor's educational need (DEN)? Should I have arranged it?)
Patient: *A breath test, I've finished my antibiotics for the bug in my stomach.*
Doctor: *How is your indigestion?*
Patient: *No problem, it's all gone now.*
Doctor: (Confused, decided to try to understand the context) *Why were you thinking you need a breath test?*
Patient: *I was reading up about the* Helicobacter *on the Internet – it said you should have a breath test after treatment.*

Understanding where the patient was coming from helped to defuse what felt like a threatening situation. However, the degree of uncertainty produced in the GP meant that it was time to look into dyspepsia again.

She has learned to say or think, 'I don't know but I'll look into it.'

The shift is not achieved easily. There follows an example of an educational workshop where another GP was helped by a simulated patient to start to grapple with the issue of learning from patients.

Vignette 7.2
A workshop took place at a conference called by the European Association for Communication in Health Care, at Warwick in September 2002 (*see* www.EACH2002.com). The method used was a well-established and validated approach used in medical and nursing education.[33–35] The workshop explored how simulated patients can best provide a patient perspective in professional learning.

A volunteer was needed who would look at a personal issue from everyday work with patients through role-play. A GP volunteered and told of a problem he had with a patient who asked him questions about aspects of her treatment provided by the hospital. He had not known the answers and had admitted this. As the patient had not returned to see him but started to see his partner instead, the GP felt he had not done this well. He reflected with the group that he often found such situations quite difficult.

In the session this was tackled in the following way: a simulated patient (SP) with considerable experience prepared a role to mirror the issue identified. She chose to role-play a patient with a history of epilepsy who wanted advice about her medication. An important aspect of this work was that the GP needed to be himself in the role-play as far as possible. So that he would not have to pretend to know the 'patient', the SP decided to role-play as a new patient. She also checked some details of the medication with another GP member of the group.

The volunteer GP then role-played a short consultation with the SP. Afterwards, the group and SP, still in role as the patient, helped the GP to discuss how the consultation had gone and to identify the many strengths in consulting that he had displayed.

These strengths included that he had carefully focused on, and responded to, the patient's concerns while exploring her present experience of epilepsy. He made the structure of the consultation transparent to the patient who was thus able to be fully involved. A lot had been discussed in less than eight minutes.

The GP then reviewed parts of the consultation that he was less sure of. He checked out how his explanation of his lack of knowledge about her medication had been received by the SP. She reassured him that it had made sense that he knew less about the details of her medication than the hospital specialist who had prescribed it. She needed to think through the effect of one of her prescribed drugs on her life and whether she should try to change it.

The GP then replayed the last part of the consultation, with feedback from the SP and suggestions from the group. He rehearsed various ways of saying what he had to offer the patient at this point. He realised that he needed to feel more comfortable about explaining where his expertise and authority lay. This was not necessarily in supplying answers to questions about specialist areas in which he was not expert. It was rather in helping the patient navigate her illness path, based on a shared exploration of her experience, on his knowledge of the possibilities in the healthcare system for information and choice, and on discussion of ways to find out more. He experimented with phrases he could use to negotiate that role and thus make his conduct of this part of the consultation equally transparent and responsive.

This example supports recent findings that clinicians need to find ways to talk differently with patients about sharing understanding and decisions about treatment.[36] As Muir Gray points out,[15] the future clinician could become a 'knowledge manager' who can:

- ask the right question and find the best answer
- help patients interpret the knowledge they have been given or have found for themselves.

WBL with a patient perspective can help professionals develop new approaches in clinical encounters with patients.

Learning from patients for wider primary care development

The changes in health access for refugees in Barnet, North London, have been discussed in *Refugees and Primary Care*.[37] These changes were brought about by local GP practices collaborating with the voluntary sector and were a direct result of the programme on preparing professionals for partnership, described earlier in this chapter.

During the programme, a practice team recognised that refugees were one group of patients whose demands felt overwhelming. They had enormous needs and the practice could not meet them. All the team – receptionists, nurses and doctors – had problems giving appropriate care. They discussed their feelings of inadequacy. They then analysed the problem.

- These patients had no records so the receptionists could not register them properly.
- As a result the nurses did not automatically perform new patient checks.
- Refugee patients had different expectations around making appointments and emergency appointments.

- Refugee patients often had more problems in their group, such as more HIV and TB, as well as post-traumatic stress disorder.
- They sometimes presented their problems in ways that the team had not previously experienced.
- Finally, communication was made harder by differences in language and culture.

The refugee patients needed quality primary healthcare which took into account their particular medical needs and communication difficulties. The doctors and nurses needed help in maintaining standards of healthcare while there was lack of knowledge, time and interpreters. The practice organisation needed to be adapted to meet these patients' needs and relieve the frustration of the team.

It became clear that many practices in Barnet had the same problems and this was an issue for the locality PCT. Extra resources for practices were needed to meet these extra problems.

Some of the organisational problems were solved by brainstorming and sharing good ideas in the project development group. Then one practice, inspired by the talk of potential for partnership, approached the local voluntary services bureau. The bureau had funding to develop work with refugees and had conducted a needs assessment. They were very pleased to be approached by health professionals. This was the first time it had happened. A local development scheme was begun: a refugee clinic has been set up at the local hospital where nurse practitioners and voluntary sector groups give advice. Voluntary groups and health professionals then gained sufficient expertise to be able to offer regular training for local practices on refugee issues. One GP reported as follows:

> It helped me to realise that feeling inadequate about my consultations with refugee patients was not just my problem. I also think I had a fantasy that I could not look after them because I didn't know enough about them. I am now clearer that they are not so different from other patients. We have to take on board their differences in the way we organise ourselves as a practice, but actually I now feel more confident that I can help them.

Involving the voluntary sector in primary care development enables frustrated professionals and needy patients to discover resources to cope with special pressures.

A matter of feelings

There is evidence that patients greatly appreciate contributing to professional learning.[38] In turn, they also understand more about the difficulties professionals face.[19] When professionals feel able to share their uncertainties with their patients, they are more comfortable and 'present' in their role. They are then more able to pay attention to patients' needs.

Professionals need support themselves to be able to give support in this way.[4,10] Professionals often stop listening and explaining in order to protect themselves from feeling their own and their patients' fears. Government and policy makers' exhortations to professionals to change tend to ignore professionals' feelings. This is not the best way to help change to happen.

Conclusion

It is clear that, in future, patients will continue to have an important role in helping primary care to develop. Their opinions of their interactions with practices are already widely canvassed, and are to be canvassed formally, by GPs, in the predicted format of GP appraisal.[39] As a result of government directives, no potential appraiser of GPs should be appointed who is not aware of the importance of the role of patients in healthcare development.

This book describes the habits and structures of WBL that enable professionals to develop their understanding and proficiency. In this chapter we have emphasised the importance of enabling the person within the patient to be heard, but also the person within the professional. We have looked at the way in which individual professionals, their primary care teams and those in a wider district can be helped to develop more sensitive and productive approaches to working with the expertise of patients and the community. Not only can this expertise be used to enhance quality of care, it can also provide invaluable support for health professionals.

References

1 Department of Health (2001) *Involving Patients and the Public in Healthcare: a discussion document.* HMSO, London.

2 Gillespie R, Florin D and Gillam S (2002) *Changing Relationships: findings of the Patient Involvement Project.* King's Fund, London.

3 Department of Health (2001) *The Expert Patient: a new approach to chronic disease management for the 21st century.* HMSO, London.

4 Salinsky J and Sackin P (2000) *What Are You Feeling, Doctor?* Radcliffe Medical Press, Oxford.

5 West L (2001) *Doctors on the Edge.* Free Association Books, London.

6 NHS Executive (2000) *Preparing Professionals for Participation with the Public.* London Regional Education Unit, London.

7   Morris P, Burton K, Reiss M *et al.* (2001) The difficult consultation. An action learning project about mental health issues in the consultation. *Ed Gen Pract.* **12**: 19–26.

8   Stewart M (1995) Effective physician–patient communication and health outcomes: a review. *Canadian Medical Association Journal.* **152**: 1423–33.

9   Campion P, Foulkes J, Neighbour R *et al.* (2002) Patient centredness in the MRCGP examination: analysis of a large cohort. *BMJ.* **325**: 691–2.

10 Morris P, Dalton E, Griffith J *et al.* (1998) Preparing for patients: preparing tomorrow's doctors. *Patient Education and Counseling.* **34**: S5–S41.

11 Maguire P and Pitkeathly C (2002) Key communication skills and how to acquire them. *BMJ.* **325**: 697–700.

12 Appleby J and Coote A (2002) *A Five-Year Health Check: a review of government health policy 1997–2002.* King's Fund, London.

13 Department of Health (2002) *Learning from Bristol: response to the Bristol Inquiry report.* Department of Health, London.

14 Coulter A (2002) *The Autonomous Patient: ending paternalism in medical care.* HMSO, London.

15 Muir Gray JA (2002) *The Resourceful Patient.* Available as an 'e-book' and in print from www.resourcefulpatient.org.

16 Fisher B, Neve H and Heritage Z (1999) Community development, user involvement and primary health care. *BMJ.* **318**: 749–50.

17 Tudor Hart J (2002) The autonomous patient: ending paternalism in medical care. *Journal of the Royal Society of Medicine.* **95**: 623–4.

18 Arntson P (1989) Improving citizens' health competencies. *Health Communication.* **1**: 29–34.

19 Morris P (1992) Citizens in health care. In: R Hambleton and M Taylor (eds) *People in Cities.* SAUS Publications, Bristol.

20 Launer J (2002) *Narrative-based Primary Care.* Radcliffe Medical Press, Oxford.

21 Tuckett D, Boulton M, Olsen C *et al.* (1985) *Meetings Between Experts: an approach to sharing ideas in medical consultations.* Tavistock, London.

22 Burton J and Morris P (2001) Mental illness or human distress? Challenges for primary care educators. *Ed Gen Pract.* **12**: 1–10.

23 Bradburn J, Fletcher G and Kennelly C (1999) *Voices in Action: training and support for lay representatives in the health service.* College of Health, London.

24 Wilson J (1999) Acknowledging the expertise of patients and their organisations. *BMJ.* **319**: 771–4.

25 Spencer J, Blackmore D, Heard S *et al.* (2000) Patient-orientated learning: a review of the role of the patient in the education of medical students. *Medical Education.* **34**: 851–7.

26 Wykurz G (1999) Patients in medical education: from passive participants to active partners. *Medical Education.* **33**: 634–6.

27 English National Board (1996) *Learning From Each Other: the involvement of people who use services and their carers in education and training.* ENB, London.

28 O'Neill F (2002) *Developing a Strategic Approach to User and Carer Involvement in Pre-registration Nursing and Midwifery Education in Leeds.* School of Healthcare Studies, Leeds.

29 Barnes D, Carpenter J and Bailey D (2000) Partnerships with service users in interprofessional education for community mental health: a case study. *J Interprofessional Care.* **14(2):** 189–200.

30 Byrne P and Long B (1976) *Doctors Talking to Patients.* HMSO, London.

31 Baker K (2001) Dramatic changes. *Br J Gen Pract.* **51:** 598–9.

32 Florin D and Coulter A (2002) Partnership in the primary care consultation. In: S Gillam and F Brooks (eds) *New Beginnings: towards patient and public involvement in primary care.* King's Fund, London.

33 Pearson A, Morris P and Whitehouse C (1985) Consumer orientated groups: a new approach to interdisciplinary teaching. *Journal of the Royal College of General Practitioners.* **35:** 381–3.

34 Morris P (1992) The development and evaluation of health education and information-giving skills for medical students and doctors. In: *Health Promotion: the role of the professional in the community.* Proceedings of a symposium. Health Promotion Research Trust, Cambridge.

35 Thistlethwaite J (2001) Learning curve. *Update.* **22 March:** 398.

36 Elwyn G, Edwards A and Kinnersley P (1999) Shared decision making in primary care: the neglected second half of the consultation. *Br J Gen Pract.* **49:** 477–82.

37 Trafford P and Winkler F (2000) *Refugees and Primary Care.* Royal College of General Practitioners, London.

38 Stacy R and Spencer J (1999) Patients as teachers: a qualitative study of patients' views on their role in a community-based undergraduate project. *Medical Education.* **33:** 688–94.

39 Greco M, Brownlea A and McGovern J (2001) Impact of patient feedback on interpersonal skills of general practice registrars: results of a longitudinal study. *Medical Education.* **35:** 748–56. Patient feedback toolkit also available from cfep@dialstart.net.

CHAPTER 8

Work based learning and poor performance

Reed Bowden and John Schofield

To be still searching what we know, not by what we know ... this is the Golden Rule ... (John Milton, 1608–1674)

Doctors whose standard of practice is consistently below an acceptable level can be difficult to identify and even more difficult to help. Many factors may influence their poor performance, including ill health, alcohol or other addictions, and stresses arising outside work. Whatever else may be required, educational advice and help will be part of the assistance offered to them. The aim will be threefold: to bring the doctor up to an acceptable level of knowledge and skills for the present needs of his or her patients; to develop or rekindle a commitment to lifelong learning; and to be ready to satisfy the educational requirements of the revalidation procedures that are about to begin.[1]

This chapter will discuss how some of the educational remediation can occur in the surgery itself.

How is poor performance made apparent?

First, it may be helpful to explain how educators become aware of these doctors, and to paint a pen-picture of a typical client.

There are two main routes of referral. The first is the local route. Until recently this was by way of health authorities (HAs), but from October 2002 the responsibility for local referral has passed to primary care trusts (PCTs). They usually have their attention drawn to the doctor through complaints from patients, staff or colleagues. Sometimes there is additional evidence from performance indicators, such as odd prescribing or rapid staff turnover. The other is the General Medical Council (GMC) route. These are doctors who have been reported to the GMC and dealt with by their Committee on Professional Performance (CPP), or occasionally by the health or conduct committees. Many of the CPP group have been through the GMC's formal assessment procedures and may have had deficiencies in knowledge and skills demonstrated objectively. The GMC puts conditions on the registration of this group of doctors, and among those conditions will be a requirement for the doctor to seek help from his Dean or Director of Postgraduate Education with his future educational needs. Sometimes these needs are listed in detail by the committee, and sometimes in outline.

Another stream of clients is made up of doctors referred to the GMC, but referred back to be helped locally without entering their formal procedures. By and large the local clients stay in their own workplaces and the educator helps them to develop a learning culture there. The GMC doctors may be allowed to return to their practices, but more often they are ordered to find a training position with a trainer or another practitioner of repute, and so they have to begin their remediation in someone else's workplace.

For the educator the most difficult task with the former group is to guarantee the quality of their educational progress, particularly for a doctor in partnership where the assessment has suggested that the whole practice is struggling. For the GMC group, the biggest problem is helping them to find a suitable placement in the first place.

We will return to both these problems, but before doing so it may help to provide a thumbnail sketch of a typical client from each category. Both doctors are presented as male, because most doctors in both groups are male. This may reflect the predominant age group, which is the fifties. There were fewer women doctors entering medical schools then. For the sake of simplicity male pronouns are used for doctors throughout this chapter.

The local route

First, a doctor coming through the local route. An immigrant doctor has been chosen in order to bring in as many factors as possible. We will return to this topic later in the chapter. This is necessarily more of a collage than a sketch, and some doctors in this category will differ from this description in many ways.

He is in his fifties and runs a single-handed inner-city practice, with a large list. For years he has struggled with his patients' problems of poverty, addiction and the demands of immigrants trying to come to terms with a new culture and a new country. Putting this alongside the routine daily grind of minor illness and the occasional major one, he has become exhausted and almost overwhelmed. He himself came to England as an immigrant many years ago, with high hopes of becoming a hospital specialist. He thought perhaps he would settle down in the UK, or he might go back home with his higher qualifications under his belt, and with a distinguished career in his own country beckoning. Somehow it didn't quite work out like that. He went through the junior grades easily enough, but when the time came to bid for the top jobs he hardly ever made the short list, and when he did the interviews went poorly. Whether the other candidates were better or whether prejudice was at work he couldn't be sure, but eventually he became discouraged and, truth to tell, a little bitter. However, there were vacancies in general practice at that time, so all was not lost. Home-grown doctors had cornered the most attractive partnerships in market towns and prosperous suburbs, but there were openings in the tougher areas, which might suit him for a couple of years.

From the outset there were unexpected problems. The premises were poky and poorly maintained. His attached staff, the midwife and health visitor, could barely provide an acceptable service in a space that was part treatment room, part consulting room and part overflow storeroom. The receptionists were loyal and did their best, often having to calm angry patients who were kept waiting too long. Eventually the pressures became too much for them and staff turnover increased. As for himself, he found he could cope with his large list if he gave a basic service, with brief consultations, liberal referrals and generous prescriptions, and didn't worry too much about screening and targets. Requests for visits were most easily dealt with by suggesting the local casualty department or a 999 call. He felt tense most of the time, and increasingly there were confrontations with patients, and sometimes shouting matches, as well as a constant dribble of complaints.

The years had gone by, and going back home was no longer an option. The children were in secondary school and there were so many ties to hold the whole family here. One thing he was proud of though, despite the difficulties at the practice; he had kept up his medical education. Every week he attended the lunchtime postgraduate sessions at the local centre. Often he was a bit late, but he'd nod to the drug reps and grab a plateful of food to eat off his lap as the speaker gave the lecture. He would have to rush off a few minutes early to get back to his antenatal clinic in time, but he did enough to get signed up. The letter came as a bolt from the blue. The health authority informed him that, in view of a number of complaints and other indicators of difficulty in providing an acceptable service, its performance advisory group would like to meet him to explore problems and suggest remedies.

The sequence of events after this point can vary from one area to another, which could give rise to allegations of uneven or unfair treatment. It is encouraging that a declared aim of the newly founded National Clinical Assessment Authority (NCAA) is to train assessors in local procedures to use nationally developed instruments, backed by the NCAA, from April 2003 onwards.[2] At the time of writing, however, the usual procedure is that a visiting team, made up of a senior member of the PCT or HA's primary care department, a GP colleague from the local medical committee (LMC) and a doctor experienced in education would come to see such a doctor at his place of work. Their visit would include inspection of the premises, interviews with the doctor and some other team members, and checks on note-keeping, prescribing and practice procedures.

They would try to be alert, in a tactful way, to the possibility of illness in the doctor, depression in particular, and might encourage the doctor towards an occupational health appointment if it seemed sensible. They would also bear in mind how other doctors in the area, with similar problems to those in the pen-picture, are coping. If all his neighbours are struggling, it would suggest that systems, rather than individuals, are at fault, or that workforce issues are behind the problem. These are the responsibility of the Commission for Health Improvement (CHI) and the Workforce Development Confederations respectively.

Those issues apart, the team would pool their findings and send a letter to the doctor setting out all their misgivings, and giving the doctor the opportunity to discuss any disputed facts and conclusions. After reaching agreement, the letter would form the basis of an action plan, listing areas for improvement and time-scales to achieve them, together with any help that might be available to bring about such improvements. One essential component of the plan would be educational advice.

The GMC route

The GMC client would have a somewhat different experience. Stripped to its essentials, it might proceed as follows.

> There were a number of complaints suggesting gross and dangerous clinical lapses; one patient had died and lack of care had been implicated. The relatives understandably expected stringent action, and the HA needed little prompting to refer this practitioner, who had been the subject of critical comment from several reliable sources for some time, to the GMC. Their screener agreed that formal assessment of the doctor's abilities using the methods available to the CPP was the correct option. The first part of this procedure involved a practice visit, along the lines of the local one, but longer and more formally structured, and with a trained lay assessor as one of the team. The team then exercised their option of recommending that he undergo the second part of the procedure, an examination of knowledge and skills using multiple choice questions (MCQs) and simulated patients and models. The results were sobering. His performance was well below the mean for the MCQs and much of the rest of the test. When the committee heard his case, the chairman told him his registration would be made conditional for a period of one year, and read out all the conditions that would apply. They are in front of him now in written form. The worst parts of the determination are listed below.

1   You may practise only in a supernumerary position attached to a recognised trainer in general practice education.
2   You must not take independent responsibility for patient care.
3   You must not take part in out-of-hours care or work for a deputising agency.

4　You are advised to seek the advice of your Dean/Director of Postgraduate Education in order to improve your medical knowledge, with particular attention to:

- prioritising your use of time
- responding to and dealing with emergencies
- chronic disease management
- prescribing
- consultation skills
- note-keeping.

At the end of one year you will be required to attend another hearing when evidence of educational progress will be expected. The committee may direct that the formal tests should be repeated.

As if all this were not bad enough, he realises that the coming year will be unpaid. Even worse, he is liable to pay the trainer and to bear any other costs of his rehabilitation.

Some characteristics are often found in both groups of clients. Denial and lack of insight are common. In the local group, it is important to stress the object of the assessment is to help the doctor and to try to prevent any possible encounters with the GMC. It helps if the existence of local resolution procedures has been well publicised in the area. The GMC group tend to dispute the committee's findings, and the educators who advise them will often find that they must first persuade the doctor that they cannot rerun the hearing or vary the terms of the determination. The doctor may dispute the objective findings of the tests despite the evidence in front of him in the comprehensive analysis of performance which he received; or the validity of the assessment may be brought into question. Its validity and reliability have, of course, been demonstrated beyond reproach.[3]

These doctors tend to be unfamiliar with the language and concepts of education, even in rudimentary form. The lunchtime lecture and the occasional evening event put on by a drug company at a local hotel are the only educational events they take part in. They are unused to the concept of self-assessment, and have no idea how to set about it. They have never been involved in audit. Reflective diaries[4] and the PUNs and DENs method[5] (discussed later) are unknown to them, and the insight required by these methods makes them hard to adopt. Significant event analysis[6] has never been tried, and nor has analysis of complaints, both of which go unrecorded anyway. They have the haziest notion of the personal development plans (PDPs) and practice professional development plans (PPDPs) which other doctors have begun to prepare.[7]

With the GMC group it will be the trainer's task to introduce these concepts, if a trainer can be found. A training practice is a learning workplace by definition. When a locally identified doctor has to improve in his own practice it falls to the Deanery educator to co-ordinate the educational input.

GMC doctors in training practices

Finding a trainer who will take on an underperforming doctor is not an easy task. Sometimes the GMC has not stipulated that the doctor supervising the client has to be a trainer, but the duties laid upon the supervising doctor are such that the skills required are seldom found in doctors without training experience. Trainers are often in short supply even for the core work of training vocational registrars, and it is not every trainer who will consider accepting an older doctor with problems. Certainly this work should not be undertaken by young and inexperienced trainers.

Sometimes it proves so difficult to find a trainer that a large part of the period of conditional registration goes past with this difficulty unresolved. When this happens, the chairman of the relevant committee may be persuaded to use his privilege to permit an approach to another doctor of repute in the educational sphere, such as an ex-trainer or a primary care tutor. It may also be necessary to ask for help from the nominated GMC caseworker over the precise meanings of some conditions. It is hard enough providing educational help without the extra responsibility of interpreting legal phrases, and risking the possibility that the arrangements, so painstakingly put together, will not be taken as acceptable when the next hearing is held.

Often the trainer's partners will have serious doubts about accepting the doctor in difficulties. There is the problem of introducing the new doctor to the patients in a neutral way. There are problems planning training for someone who has restrictions placed on their involvement in care, prescribing and on-call commitments. The usual duty of 'logging and mapping' training encounters takes on increased importance, as the evidence will be required by the GMC at the next committee hearing, and the questioning of the trainer can be rigorous. It is essential that the client doctor makes the whole GMC dossier available to the trainer at the outset, as occasionally trainers have found themselves being questioned on documents that they had not seen before the day of the hearing.

When trying to help a doctor who cannot engage fully in clinical care, the trainer must modify the learning experience. Joint surgeries, which have a limited role in the early weeks of training for most vocational registrars, assume greater importance. Later the client can be introduced to video-recordings of himself in consultation, and how to analyse and improve consulting skills. This requires full patient consent of course. In parallel with this, the trainer will teach self-assessment methods and demonstrate the range of resources that the client can tap into to fulfil the learning needs. Another area of work which becomes more important in these circumstances is audit activity. Few clients will have had any experience in this field, and introducing them to it provides insights into clinical care, service provision, teamwork and quality assurance, all aspects of practice which tend to be among their weak points. Audit is also a revalidation requirement, so familiarity with the technique will have lasting benefits.

The supervising trainer needs to have well-developed pastoral skills. The client will be demoralised and possibly bitter, and to make good his deficiencies and rebuild self-respect is a delicate task. In particular, there may be financial problems. Time spent retraining is unpaid, nor is there any obligation on Deaneries to fund the trainer, except for the rare client who has been under the Health Committee. This means that the client and the trainer must agree the trainer's remuneration between them. Their deliberations may take the standard training grant as a starting point, but the decision is theirs alone. It is sensible for them to draw up a simple contract covering training and learning obligations and financial matters.

The trainer will need to consider how he can demonstrate progress in the attached doctor. A simple answer is to use the modules of summative assessment.[8] This process was designed for new entrants to general practice, but adapts well for underperformers and is sometimes stipulated as an assessment method by the GMC. Deaneries are able to enter the client doctor into the process using special codes that exclude these submissions from the statistical analysis of the new entrants' performance. Video and audit submissions are dealt with at first level only. The extra work and expense generated for the Deanery is very small.

It is important to ensure, as the date for the next hearing approaches, that all specific points in the conditions have been covered. For example, the fictional determination above included comments on note-keeping, which frequently happens in real life. The committee would wish to hear that the doctor understood why good notes matter for good care, how they help other doctors who may take over care, their usefulness in learning and teaching and so on; and also that he was now writing sensible, legible notes or, in the case of a fully computerised practice, entering properly coded headings with appropriate extra text.

At the hearing, if the trainer and the adviser involved are not convinced that enough progress has been made, they should not feel inhibited about expressing their wish that the committee should exercise its option to ask the doctor to take the formal assessment again.

Locally referred doctors: turning the surgery into a learning workplace

Many elements go into making a workplace an efficient learning environment. Some can be influenced directly by an educational adviser, and others require liaison with colleagues whose skills and resources are different.

- Is the working environment calm and orderly?
- Is it adequately staffed?
- Are the list size and practice area compatible with good practice?

- Does the workload allow for continuing education as an integral part of the working week?
- Do established systems, where present, work?
- Is there advice and help available from the PCT or HA?
- Can the necessary educational remedies be applied there?

Is it calm and orderly?

Good work can be done in dismal premises, and poor work can come out of attractive premises. Most often chaos reigns in the practice of the underperforming doctor, and the adviser may feel that a great deal of good could be done with a small skip and a couple of hours of vigorous rearrangement. It may be best to put these feelings to one side, however, and to advise gradual change, in consultation with HA colleagues, particularly as their specialist knowledge of health and safety legislation will be needed. The HA colleague will also know whether any grants are available for extending or redecoration, or even whether relocation may be on the cards.

Sometimes small changes can have a marked effect. One practice put its receptionists behind grilles to protect them from physical intimidation by patients. When the grilles came down, threats evaporated. Colour matters; dark blue, the colour of depression and putrefaction, and dark green, the colour of public lavatories and army lorries, should perhaps be avoided in waiting rooms and consulting rooms.

Is it adequately staffed?

Are the list size and practice area compatible with good practice?

Typically an underperforming doctor will have a big list and offer a basic service helped by a small staff. He may resist changes on the grounds that income will fall if he works any other way, and those who help him may have to demonstrate that this does not necessarily follow. An average list can often generate the same income, provided a full service is given and no items attracting payment are missed. A good practice manager will keep on top of this. Additional staff, a practice nurse for example, may often generate income in excess of her own wages.

The PCT can offer advice on drawing the practice boundary and sending out letters to those patients living outside it and who will need to register elsewhere.

The PCT or HA can also be invaluable in advising on appointments to key positions, perhaps by persuading the doctor to let one of their senior people sit in on appointments interviews, or by suggesting short-term attachments in key posts while newer staff settle in. The hope is that providing a rounded service to a smaller clientele will not only bring greater professional satisfaction but also allow time for reflection and study.

Education as part of the working week

Traditionally our continuing education has taken place outside our regular clinical work, and the prime movers in providing it have been drug companies, who cannot be regarded as disinterested. However, the episodes from which we can learn most tend to occur in the working week, and within consultations. We can learn from consultations that go well, and perhaps more from those that go badly. Then there are consultations where we are stumped for a diagnosis, or where patients require information and we are unsure what to say or who to call on for help.

Apart from consultations, our core work provides other learning opportunities. If a patient makes a complaint, is this recorded as it should be and is the justice or otherwise of the complaint given fair consideration? From time to time there will be unexpected significant events: new diagnoses of malignancy, including some where we would hope that screening procedures would offer an early warning; new infarcts and strokes; premature deaths; and obstetric catastrophes.

Employed and attached staff see our patients from a different angle and have a different body of knowledge about them; but do we make the opportunities to get together with the other team members and complete the jigsaw?

Audit, that rather dreary word that doctors stole from accountants, offers insights of all kinds into our working practices.

The problem is that it takes insight to benefit from all this educational raw material, and insight is a commodity that is often in short supply among doctors who underperform. It also takes time, though often less time than one would think at first.

Educators who work with underperforming doctors have a propaganda battle on their hands to get this point across. This work at a personal level is being mirrored by our negotiators at a national level, making the point to the government that a constantly re-educated workforce means factoring in protected time for learning. Some PCTs have shown the way by arranging study sessions, usually of half a day, for all the practices in their area, for subjects of broad interest across a district. There is only emergency cover while the session is going on.

Do established systems, where present, work?

The disorganisation which characterises dysfunctional practices is often most marked in practice systems.

Repeat prescribing is usually muddled, which implies danger to patients. Often the practice has not moved to computer based repeat prescribing, and staff have to try to cope with handwritten lists of drugs on cards stuffed into record envelopes. Faced with demands for 'the big red pills' or 'the ones for my breathing' it is little wonder that they can develop high levels of stress over this issue. Often the confusion is compounded by a lack of any review policy, and there may also be illegal practices, such as pre-signed prescriptions for receptionists to complete.

Complaints are rarely recorded. Often it is established that verbal complaints are frequent, and it is true that most of these will never proceed to written form, but a totally blank complaints book, if indeed there is a book, strains belief.

More basic systems, such as appointments or simply attendance, can be rudimentary.

It is rare to find a system for dealing with in-surgery emergencies such as collapse or anaphylactic shock. There is no emergency tray, or if there is, it is locked away and there has been no staff training in what to do if someone needs life support.

Staff are neglected in other ways too. It is unusual to find systematic pay reviews and there are often no job descriptions and sometimes no contracts. Appraisal is unknown, and opportunities for staff education for their own career advancement are absent. In a nutshell, they are just left to get on with it.

Is there advice and help available from the PCT or HA?

The answer is always yes, but the amount varies, and so does the enthusiasm with which it is offered. It is important to remember that these doctors or partnerships have often acquired a degree of notoriety locally. We all have heartsink patients, and these are the heartsink practices which have been making HA officers groan for years. The difference now is that we are moving towards formal systems of assessment and remediation which require substantiated evidence, and which are meant to be well advertised, transparent and, above all, helpful rather than punitive. With the reorganisation of HAs, more of the advice and help will come from the clinical governance committees of PCTs, and indeed the Health Act of 1999 has made them responsible for providing a 'quality service'.[9] Some ways of providing help have been referred to in the preceding paragraphs. Help with premises should be emphasised again, as transformations in attitude and performance have occasionally followed moving to better premises or the major refurbishment of the existing accommodation. Help with staffing has been mentioned. Some PCTs are beginning to employ doctors for duties wherever they may be needed across an area, and it may prove a steadying influence for one of these doctors to help out while problems are addressed. The practice manager has a key role. If the PCT can help to find the right person for this job, a great number of staff problems begin to improve.

Much can be done to improve systems, especially with help from the prescribing adviser. Not only can the clarity of intention, and the procedures for issuing drugs and arranging follow-up procedures improve, but there is scope for influencing overprescribing and bizarre prescribing if these are present, and increasing the proportion of generic prescriptions. It is almost learning and teaching by stealth.

Some would say that reorganising prescribing is an ideal opportunity to push for computerisation if the practice has not yet made this move, or to expand it if it has. This is often so. It is pointless to suggest a new paper based system for a process that cries out for a computer; however, a new computer system can be stressful, and more so when many changes are being made to a practice. It may be kinder to cross that bridge later. A crucial function of the PCT representative is to liaise with the educator, and sometimes with an LMC colleague, to see that the doctor is progressing in accordance with the action plan as time goes on. It may be a year or more before the formal supervision comes to an end, and even then the PCT will need to be reassured that the doctor or practice remains fully involved in all clinical governance initiatives.

It may also be possible to offer the opportunity of visiting other practices to pick up ideas, or even to suggest a 'buddy system' for mutual support. These networks are often best developed among team members other than the doctors. Many areas have practice manager groups. Some PCTs have a designated officer whose remit is to search out helpful innovations from all their practices and encourage others to use them.

Assuming that all this effort produces an environment in which education can flourish, there remains the final consideration, which involves the educational adviser more than anybody.

Can the necessary educational remedies be applied there?

We have agreed that in a learning workplace a doctor learns from his patients, from his partners if he has any, from his staff and from various written sources, such as complaints, the critical events log, and prescribing analyses and cost (PACT) data.

Consultations are the richest source of educational opportunity, and this is a group of doctors in whom communication difficulties are often assessed as poor, so this makes a good starting place.

The educator will want to introduce the client to one of the established ways of analysing the consultation, for him to study away from the practice. Many such ways exist.[10] All tend to share the headings of: welcome, dealing with main problem, allowing time for subsidiary problems, suggesting management plans, agreeing a suitable plan and farewell. The trick is to apply the system throughout each consultation, and this group of doctors will need help here. One way is for the adviser to sit in as an observer; another is to use a video camera. Both ways are open to the criticism that they alter the dynamic of the consultation, though this effect seems to wear off quite quickly. If sitting-in is used, the adviser may ask a communication skills specialist to help with this. The specialist will have more experience and can offer ongoing support in the practice as needed. With videos, there is a limit to how much can be gained by the doctor viewing them alone. It is more helpful to let a colleague with experience look through them and advise accordingly. An experienced trainer, not necessarily from the immediate area, a summative assessment video assessor or an MRCGP video assessor would be ideal.

If the room layout makes video impossible, there may be something to be gained from an audio recording. In either case, written patient consent, before and after, is essential.

Some consultations end without fulfilling the patient's need because the doctor does not know or has forgotten the information that would bring about a successful outcome. The ending is fudged in some way, or a referral is made. Provided the doctor has the insight to spot these consultations, and the presence of mind to note down the area of deficiency, these patients' unmet needs (PUNs) can provide a valuable spur to learning by indicating the doctor's educational needs (DENs). This is the essence of the PUNs and DENs method. It is an example of self-assessment of learning needs, an area which is difficult for most of us and usually quite novel to underperforming colleagues.

Practice meetings offer educational opportunities, as well as the chance to refresh the memory concerning the complementary roles of other team members and to discuss specific patients who are causing concern to more than one team member. Some education may be undertaken together. Basic life support, for instance, could bring in all staff, medical or otherwise. Not only does this kind of exercise have potential value for the patients, but it is important in bonding a team and showing that all its members are valued.

It is important to advise the doctor to keep a record of all educational activity inside the practice. With PUNs and DENs for example, or critical event analysis, there should be a note of the learning need identified, together with the learning activity it gave rise to. Reports from the communication skills adviser, or any outside adviser, should be requested and kept in a learning portfolio with certificates of educational events attended outside the practice.[11]

The benefits of audit have been mentioned.[12] It helps, before embarking on an audit, to seek advice from an experienced colleague. The first and best piece of advice will be to keep it short and simple (the KISS acronym). The scrutiny of one small part of the service on offer, and its measurement against justified criteria, form the first part of the work. If, as usually happens, the practice is not reaching the standard it has set for itself, then changes should be put in place and their effect should be checked after an interval.

Finally, there are educational advantages in completing a PDP and PPDP. There are a number of outline proformas to choose from, often accessible from Deanery websites. All of them make the doctor pause and reflect on his present situation, his future ambitions and the possible stepping-stones from now to then. Most also have spaces for logging educational activities, and they are an important part of the documentation required for revalidation appraisals and the five-yearly revalidation itself.

Maximising the effect of the remedies: how can educational theory help?

The prime responsibility of the educator is patient safety. It is easy to become so wrapped up in the helping process with the doctor concerned that one forgets that he is not the final customer of the whole exercise, but an intermediary in the delivery of a service.[13]

We have discussed the importance of excluding illness as a cause of underperformance. If the educator is not confident that that has been done, it is important to urge the client to see his own doctor or use the occupational health service.

Even with illness ruled out, all these doctors are, in a sense, bereaved. They have lost status in the community, and taken knocks to their self-esteem and their finances. The well-known concomitants of bereavement, denial, guilt, disbelief and anger will all be present in varying proportions.[14] The timescale to rebuild their lives must be realistic and achievable.

The educator may doubt whether the doctor is retrainable, either on grounds of his attitude or the sheer range of deficiencies which have been demonstrated. When the referral comes from the GMC, that decision has been made by other people, and the adviser has to make the best of it. With local referrals, it may be necessary to suggest to the practice support group that referral to the GMC may be the better option. If the adviser hears of the case early enough, he may urge referral to the NCAA, one of whose prime aims is to decide which level of involvement is most appropriate.

One problem is that no one can be sure whether the doctors under discussion are at the lowest part of a Gaussian distribution of competence or whether they are intrinsically different.[15] Quite often there is anecdotal evidence from colleagues who knew these doctors years earlier, at medical school or elsewhere, that they always had odd attitudes or were always distinct in some unflattering way. If this holds true for most underperformers, then the attitude tests which some medical schools are introducing for their applicants should be applauded.

Doctors who trained abroad, as in the first pen-picture, are over-represented in underperformance procedures, which raises several questions. It may be too late to speculate on the quality of their basic medical education, but not too late to hope that the reciprocal arrangements for recognising degrees would be more reliable today. Not only is there the question of educational quality, but also of style. If their educational experience has all been of a didactic and rigid nature it requires a superhuman effort to adapt to new concepts like self-assessment and problem based learning, especially well on in life. Then there is the matter of transcultural training to help them fit into British medicine, which is on offer to immigrant doctors now but did not happen before. The miracle is that so many immigrant doctors, subject as they were to all the difficulties listed in the first pen-picture, have managed to provide such a high quality service in some very tough areas. Perhaps we should not miss the opportunity to consider what extent racism, overt, covert or institutionalised, is implicated in underperformance work. It was suggested earlier, in the first pen-picture, that unfair pressure may have resulted in this doctor finding himself in a difficult practice. There is also a widespread feeling, though unsupported by hard evidence, that white doctors are less likely to be called to account for persistent underperformance than doctors from other racial groups.

The RCGP likes to celebrate the best in general practice, and make it better. This is laudable in a Royal College, but it raises the question of how this affects the less able. Would the quality of the profession as a whole improve more if the biggest effort went into helping the strugglers? Put simplistically, if underperformers are a breed apart then they should find careers outside medicine, and if they're not, then we have a system failure to put right. Perhaps these issues will be considered by the promised NHSU.[16]

When remediation is going ahead in a practice, very few of the educational methods that can be applied are amenable to objective assessment. Unobserved casework clearly is not, and neither are methods that require insight and reflection, such as PUNs and DENs. Video-recorded work and audit get closer to objectivity. It may be possible to use statistical process control to see whether abilities are improving.[17]

Casework and its derivatives may be difficult to assess, but they have the advantage of being patient centred and problem based, which are the bedrock of modern medical education.[18]

The adviser has the advantage of basing his help on a knowledge of assessed deficiencies. This permits a degree of 'just-for-you' tailoring of the help offered.[19] Pressing and immediate needs are dealt with first, the 'just-in-time' philosophy.[20]

Encouraging a colleague to make his workplace a learning workplace does not mean that out-of-house education is of little importance. Indeed, it has advantages. The responsibility of patient care is lifted, and educational challenges can be put forward with safety. There is the stimulation of learning with others, and it is efficient in terms of cost and trainer time. With some skills, minor surgery for example, the benefits are obvious. A combination of learning venues works best. We all have a duty to demonstrate our commitment to keeping our skills and competence up to date.[16] If an adviser can help his colleague to develop that commitment, his job is well done indeed.

Underperformance work and quality assurance

The climate in healthcare is moving towards a guaranteed quality of care to our patients, and so the assessment and upgrading of doctors is a priority. From an industrial viewpoint the importance of *training on the job*[21] was one of the guiding principles of continuous quality improvement (CQI). The other significant movements are the change to the team approach and the focus on the needs of the customer. There is a great opportunity here to involve other members of the primary care team in improved working practices and joint training sessions. As mentioned earlier, it is common practice now to have closedown afternoons in general practice where the calls are taken by an agency. In such an atmosphere, the use of a facilitator to work on joint care protocols, patient management procedures, etc., could well move the whole practice forward. It may seem a cliché to say, 'work smarter not harder', but this is what we are aiming at. The potential release of the abilities and imagination of the reception staff, managers, nurses and other team members should more than offset the training time involved.

One of the most neglected resources is the patients themselves. It is really surprising sometimes when patients are asked how things could be improved, to find that they come up with very insightful suggestions. To quote from the *Harvard Business Review*: *'It seems clear, then, that effective learning depends on the availability of peers and their willingness to act as mentors and coaches'.*[22] We believe that the use of these mentors to assist doctors experiencing problems is both vital to the safety of patients and cost-effective to the country at large.

References

1 The General Medical Council website: www.gmc-org/revalidation.

2 NCAA (2002) NCAA *Handbook for Prototype Phase: general practice in England, information for PCTs*. www.ncaa.nhs.uk.

3 Southgate L (ed.) (2001) The GMC's performance procedures: a study of their implementation and impact. *Medical Education.* **35**: supplement 1.

4   Al-Shehri A (1995) Learning by reflection in general practice: a study report. *Ed Gen Pract.* **7**: 237–48.

5   Eve R (2000) Learning with PUNs and DENs – a method for determining educational needs and the evaluation of its use in primary care. *Ed Gen Pract.* **11**: 73–9.

6   Pringle M (1999) Significant event auditing. In: T van Zwanenberg and J Harrison (eds) *Clinical Governance in Primary Care.* Radcliffe Medical Press, Oxford.

7   Rughani A (2000) *The GP's Guide to Personal Development Plans.* Radcliffe Medical Press, Oxford.

8   Bowden R and Jackson N (2002) The principles of assessment. In: Y Carter and N Jackson (eds) *Guide to Education and Training for Primary Care.* Oxford University Press, Oxford.

9   Department of Health (1999) *Health Act 1999*, section 18. HMSO, London.

10 Tate P (2000) *MRCGP: preparing and passing.* Royal Society of Medicine Press, London.

11 Snadden D and Thomas M (1998) The use of portfolio learning in medical education. *Medical Teacher.* **20**: 192–9.

12 Bowie P, Garvie A, Oliver J *et al.* (2002) Impact on non-principals in general practice of the summative assessment audit project. *Ed Primary Care.* **13**: 356–61.

13 Sallis E (1996) *The Role of the Consumer in Quality. Total quality management in education.* Kogan Page, London.

14 Parkes CM (1998) Coping with loss: facing loss. *BMJ.* **316**: 1521–4.

15 Pell AR (1995) *Examining the Trait Based Appraisal System. The complete idiot's guide to managing people.* Alpha Books, Indianapolis, IN.

16 Department of Health (2001) *Working Together, Learning Together – a framework for life-long learning for the NHS.* HMSO, London.

17 Slack N, Chambers S, Harland C *et al.* (1998) *Operations Management.* Financial Times, Pitman Publishing, London.

18 Neufeld VR, Woodward CA and Macleod SM (1989) The MacMaster MD Programme: a case study of renewal in medical education. *Acad Med.* **64**: 423–32.

19 Gower SEA (1996) The really useful handbook for the practice receptionist. *BMJ.* **313**: 1091.

20 Monden Y (1998) *Toyota Production System. An integrated approach to just-in-time.* EMP Books, Norcross, GA.

21 Deming WE (1982) *Institute Training. Out of crisis.* MIT, Cambridge, MA.

22 Wenger EC and Snyder WM (2001) The Organizational Frontier. *Harvard Business Review on Organizational Learning.* Harvard Business School Press, Boston, MA.

CHAPTER 9

Work based learning and clinical governance

John Toby

Background

Much of this book looks at the meaning and methods of learning, especially in the workplace. This chapter is an exploration of the relationship between clinical governance and learning. It is not a textbook on clinical governance, which now has a large literature of its own. However, a brief review reveals the closeness of the relationship and the unique contributions that each can make to the other.

Clinical governance has its origins in the pursuit of quality, which has lain close to the heart of medical education since its earliest days.[1] As medicine and society have become more complex, so has the difficulty in defining quality. The work of Donabedian and Maxwell, among others, in the 1970s and 1980s helped to define a multifaceted approach to quality which has increasingly included accountability as an explicit feature.[2,3] The drawing together of much of this thought into an organisational arrangement alongside the provisions for corporate governance is having a profound effect on the NHS. The original description of clinical governance was as:

> *A framework through which NHS organisations are accountable for continually improving the quality of their services and safeguarding high standards of care by creating an environment in which excellence in clinical care will flourish.*[4]

Government publications and legislation have made it clear that clinical governance is a key part of the philosophy and practice of the NHS.[5–7] It therefore represents a fundamental change from the time when quality initiatives may have been seen as an optional extra and when individual studies were often carried out on a project basis.[8]

Clinical governance was adopted with some enthusiasm by those working in the NHS because it offered a welcome change of emphasis away from financial drivers and towards improvements in patient care. It also offered the possibility of focusing on the conditions needed for the professional development required for those improvements.

In reality, clinical governance wears at least two faces – a sterner face of governance and a gentler face of support. The governance face is more narrowly defined and principally concerns quality assurance, which is a process that demonstrates and confirms the quality of care. The supportive aspects are wider, embracing in addition the mechanisms and environment needed to improve quality. Both quality assurance and quality improvement also have their own extensive literatures in health and in the wider world of work. The implementation of clinical governance may be hampered by a failure to reconcile these two aspects. While the current trend is to focus on the developmental aspects, this may leave expectations of quality assurance unsatisfied.[9]

There is a second way in which clinical governance has two faces. Some aspects are more capable of precise definition and measurement, while others are qualitative and require a greater degree of judgement. There is a tendency to set these two characteristics in opposition, creating conflicts and polarities where none are necessary. Rather, a mature approach to quality requires the use of a wide variety of methods of evaluation.

There is yet another way in which clinical governance may be two-faced. It may serve the quality agenda identified by patients and professionals or it may serve to confirm the achievement of arbitrary targets which do not necessarily reflect the long-term interests of patients or the NHS. It is inevitable that both those with short-term and those with long-term agendas will seek to use data to support their arguments. It is important that people with predominantly long-term and developmental agendas are not discouraged from using the opportunities presented by clinical governance both to demonstrate improvements in care and to inform education for the future.

It is also important that semantic and politically motivated dispute is not allowed to detract from the value of clinical governance as a vehicle for quality improvement and professional development. Finally, it should be remembered that, when introduced to the NHS, clinical governance was seen as a ten-year programme.[7] This is only now at around its mid-point.

Clinical governance therefore embraces many of the aspirations of the professions involved in the delivery of care, their dilemmas and the ways in which these may be addressed. Its elements have great potential as positive forces for the development of services for patients and for the professional development of individuals. Many of the drivers for clinical governance may seem to derive from the recent problems of the medical profession but most of its real potential is in quality improvement and education.

The relationship with education

This potential for supporting professional development makes clinical governance a central focus for education, especially in the workplace where many of its practical applications lie.

An earlier analysis identified the potential for WBL to provide both evidence of learning needs and also opportunities for learning.[10] Clinical governance provides an excellent example of this principle. On the one hand, learners will find that they may need to acquire new knowledge, skills and attitudes to participate in clinical governance. On the other hand, it offers enormous opportunities for learning. Clinical governance and learning are inextricably linked in theory as well as in practice.

Individual learning has been shown to be a cyclical process. Similarly a cyclical process underlies quality improvement. This process is akin to a form of corporate learning. It has been described in other parts of this book which cover collaborative and team learning (Chapters 1–4) and clinical effectiveness (Chapter 10). Clinical governance offers the opportunity to practise newly acquired skills on which individual learning depends and from which quality improvement results. The central role of education to clinical governance is also recognised by those who work to promote and develop the latter.[11]

All of the techniques of clinical governance offer learning opportunities in the workplace. However, clinical governance also requires and creates an attitude of supportive challenge that characterises both effective deliverers of service and learning organisations. It is in this less tangible but more important way that the synergy between clinical governance and WBL is most apparent.

The place of clinical governance in learning can be explored in a number of different ways:

- as a fundamental building block for patient care
- as a support for lifelong learning and personal development
- as a series of components providing tools for professional development
- as a subject which creates its own learning needs.

This chapter focuses on the contribution that clinical governance makes to learning rather than the learning needs that it creates, although individual readers may identify these in passing.

A building block for patient care

Clinical governance represents the current consensus and embraces some of the divergent opinions about the provision of high quality care within the setting of a diverse society. All people working within the NHS will be exposed to the many pressures that arise from the pursuit of quality in all its dimensions. Without some familiarity with the issues and acceptance of their relevance, clinicians may find themselves increasingly uncomfortable in their professional roles. An early exploration of these issues thus provides an essential foundation for learning clinical practice in the NHS in the 21st century.

This is not to suggest that either the concepts or content of clinical governance are likely to remain constant. However, it is only from an understanding of the present that clinicians will be able to make sense of the world of healthcare as it evolves.

A support for lifelong learning and professional development

The framework of clinical governance allows clinicians to organise their continuing learning and to assemble evidence to review their learning needs and to demonstrate their quality. Thus the direct linkage between clinical governance and learning will continue to be emphasised through appraisal which will use data from clinical practice to inform the process. In its turn evidence of satisfactory appraisal will be a major component of what will be needed for the revalidation of medical practitioners.[12] Personal development plans will increasingly focus learning on the areas needed to improve service delivery, although these should be interpreted in a broad way to allow for rounded personal development rather than simply the acquisition of individual skills.

Components for professional development

There is a need for a framework or a number of frameworks to give a structure to learning in any setting. While this must not be too intrusive and must be sensitive to the individual learner, it must provide a map and also ensure that what needs to be learned is learned. Clinical governance provides just such a framework for the clinical and organisational aspects of service delivery to sit alongside the frameworks for effective learning set out in other chapters of this book.

There are many descriptions of the components of clinical governance, but most include those in Box 9.1. A brief look at each of these will show how fundamental they are to the core functions of the clinical professions and the satisfactory functioning of individuals. It is not the intention of this chapter to explore these areas in detail but to illustrate the scope and the potential for learning.

> **Box 9.1:** Components of clinical governance
>
> - Clinical effectiveness.
> - Patient and public involvement.
> - Organisation.
> - Significant event audit.
> - Risk management.
> - Clinical ethics.
> - Clinical audit.

Clinical effectiveness

Clinicians will identify a number of tools from the repertoire of evidence based medicine that support clinical effectiveness in practice and which are described in Chapter 10. These include guidance from the National Institute for Clinical Excellence and from many national bodies, National Service Frameworks, and a wide variety of trials and other information from the literature. While their applications are not limited to the workplace, it is there that the interface between what may be theoretically desirable and what is practicable is seen in its sharpest relief. The conflicts between theory and practice, between universal guidelines and individual patient choice, between the desirable and the affordable are played out on a day-to-day basis.

Patient participation

Clinical governance is one of the areas of healthcare in which the involvement of patients is increasing and this influence enriches its potential for learning. As with clinical governance itself, patient and public involvement provides both a source of learning and a topic for which learners will need to prepare.

The involvement of patients in clinical governance can be at a number of levels. These include setting its directions at national and local level and its application in the processes of review and education. At the local level, different primary care organisations and individual practices are evolving different approaches and moving at different paces – therefore they will offer different learning opportunities. However, the possibilities include:

- methods of patient and public involvement
- awareness of the key elements of patient satisfaction and their measurement
- the value and management of suggestions and complaints.

Within the local organisation there should be opportunities to join in and to observe the work of patients in groups developing approaches to clinical governance.

Many practices are involving groups of patients to help with general developments – often in the form of patient participation groups or in the development of specific services such as the care of people with specific conditions.

As important, these various possibilities offer the potential to question the objectives of involving patients and to learn from them. The opportunities range from deepening understanding of individual clinical conditions, seeing the arrangements for care from patient perspectives, to questioning priorities in one's own approaches and the NHS as a whole.

Organisation

The organisation of healthcare is often a dry subject. It comes to life when it is considered as part of the patients' pathways through the system and especially when these may be causing problems. Clinical governance thus provides a way of studying organisation and management that is led by clinical quality and the care of patients.

Working and learning in teams are at the heart of clinical governance. Again the direct study of such arrangements may seem to lack relevance, but they can be appreciated in the context of specific patients or disease management. These therefore provide a setting in which to both discuss and experience this and to help refine strategies for making the best use of the opportunities.

A key element of WBL is the support of peers. Participation in the activity of a group is a motivator and most of us need a little help with motivation from time to time. Members of a group are also a support in times of difficulty. Individual members of a group bring different perspectives, and where these come from different disciplines the resulting discussions are much deeper. The place of interdisciplinary activities is unclear in much of education but in continuing professional development, especially in general practice, it is well established.

Significant event audit

The study of cases and situations that seem to have potentially or actually important consequences has always been a source of learning. It is worth pointing out that such situations may be sources of pride as well as of concern. The ability to manage such discussions is one test of an effective organisation and will be closely allied with its ability to deal with complaints in a constructive way. The study of significant events has now been systematised to enable the maximum learning to be obtained.[13]

Risk management

This has emerged as a key element of clinical governance. As with other elements, its components are not new but their collection together has given new emphasis to their importance. It brings together clinical and non-clinical risk and embraces also the management of complaints and suggestions from patients, users and carers.

Clinical ethics

It is not possible to have many discussions within the areas of clinical governance without stumbling on ethical issues. These may involve dilemmas such as those posed by accountability, the allocation of resources including time, and judging acceptable degrees of risk. This ethical component enriches discussions and extends the potential for learning, especially where a patient or public perspective can be included.

Clinical audit

A key component of clinical governance is clinical audit, which needs to be a planned, systematic and continuing review of important clinical areas. While most practices have been carrying out audits for some time, it is only now that this regular review has become a regular part of the organisations.

Requirements for clinical governance

Clinical governance needs an infrastructure including:

- high quality data
- information technology
- educational opportunities
- organisational support.

These also provide learning opportunities because each has its own set of knowledge and skills. While some of the details of these do not need to be part of the learning for all clinicians, there are some that are essential learning for the provision of good quality care and for leadership roles.

Jennifer had recently started as a GP registrar. She had been working in a medical department in hospital prior to this and she was horrified to find that a number of patients with a recorded high blood pressure were either being treated inadequately or were not on treatment. She was being encouraged to undertake some project work and this seemed to offer her a suitable topic. Her immediate thought was to improve her knowledge of the guidelines on the treatment of hypertension, audit the practice patients and present the findings to persuade the practice to do better. Her trainer encouraged her to reflect on the wider determinants of high quality practice and, in particular, to explore the areas covered by clinical governance before deciding on the best focus for her work. On reflection, she realised that although her knowledge, and that of the practice, of the guidelines on the management of hypertension could be improved, this was unlikely to be the major reason for the problem she had identified.

Jennifer was encouraged to set up a small working group involving a practice nurse, a receptionist, a member of the administrative staff, a patient suggested by the local PCT and a GP. An audit quickly confirmed the unsatisfactory state of affairs and possible contributory factors were considered. While lack of knowledge about clinical management was one, the most likely candidates for change included use of the computer system by clinicians and staff, an administrative system to reduce the number of patients falling through the net and the provision of information for patients both verbally and in writing. It was agreed that there would be a full team meeting (which would also review the guidelines) and that improved arrangements were required for the monitoring of patients. It was also clear that the practice needed a way to involve its own patients in giving advice and a separate discussion about patient participation was begun.

In the course of this project, Jennifer found that her knowledge of hypertension had improved slightly from its initial high level but that she had acquired insights into the work of clinical and non-clinical staff, and had learned a great deal about the problems of getting and using high quality data. She had enjoyed working with the small team which she had led and had been able to explore the contribution that patients can make to their own care and the running of the practice.

Conclusion

It is clear, then, that clinical governance and work based learning are inextricably linked. In order to deliver service of a high quality we must be patient centred, looking outward and objectively at the evidence of the quality of our care. We must also be reflective, seeking to match what we do, both as individuals and in teams, to the best possible standards. By so doing, we will continue to be made aware of our own needs as learners. In the past, some clinical subjects, such as syphilis and diabetes, have been proposed as being of such breadth as to encompass the whole of what needs to be learned to practise medicine.

In the context of the NHS at the beginning of the 21st century, clinical governance may fulfil such a role for those providing care in multidisciplinary teams.

The association of clinical governance with enjoyment is not necessarily an obvious one and yet many general practices and clinical departments enjoy multidisciplinary discussions based on clinical topics. The chemistry provided by focusing on the care of patients, effective teamworking and well-applied clinical science remains a strong attraction despite the many pressures in the system. It is also a self-fulfilling activity since the practice of regular meetings devoted to quality improvement is one of the surest guarantees that this will occur. To be involved in these occasions as a learner will demonstrate the value of clinical governance better than any book.

References

1   Jones WHS (1923) *Hippocrates*. Heinemann, London.

2   Donabedian A (1980) *Explorations in Quality Assessment and Monitoring*. Health Administration Press, Ann Arbor, MI.

3   Maxwell RJ (1984) Quality assessment in health. *BMJ*. **288**: 1470–2.

4   Scally G and Donaldson LJ (1998) Clinical governance and the drive for quality improvement in the new NHS in England. *BMJ*. **317**: 61–5.

5   Department of Health (1997) *The New NHS – modern, dependable*. HMSO, London.

6   Department of Health (1999) *Clinical Governance: quality in the new NHS*. Health Service Commissioner 1999/065. HMSO, London.

7   Secretary of State for Health (2000) *NHS Plan – a plan for investment, a plan for reform*. Department of Health, London.

8   Kazandijan V (2002) Can the sum of projects end up in a program? *Qual Saf Health Care*. **11**: 212–13.

9   Campbell S, Sheaff R, Sibbald B *et al.* (2002) Implementing clinical governance in English primary care groups/trusts. *Qual Saf Health Care*. **11**: 9–14.

10 Seagraves L, Osborne N, Neal P *et al.* (1996) *Learning in Smaller Companies – final report*. University of Stirling, Stirling.

11 Clark C and Smith L (2002) Clinical governance and education. *Br J Clinical Governance*. **7**: 261–6.

12 Bradley T (2002) Integrating appraisal, revalidation and PDPs. *Practitioner*. **246**: 543–6.

13 Pringle M, Bradley C, Carmichael C *et al.* (1995) *Significant Event Auditing*. Occasional Paper 70. RCGP, London.

CHAPTER 10

Clinical effectiveness: integrating effective practice into daily life

Yvonne Carter and Maggie Falshaw

Knowledge is of two kinds. We know a subject ourselves, or we know where we can find information upon it. (Samuel Johnson, 1775)

Introduction

This chapter looks at some ways that work based learning can be used by primary care workers in their attempts to put evidence into daily practice. The chapter has an overview of the development of evidence based medicine (EBM) in the later 20th century and its incorporation into clinical practice through both national and local strategies.

There is no place in the modern NHS for the piecemeal adoption of unproven therapies, or for hanging on to outdated, ineffective treatments.[1]

This statement, from *A First Class Service*, outlines the government's commitment to the development and implementation of evidence based healthcare in the National Health Service. Evidence based healthcare has been widely adopted in the UK in the last decade. This can be seen in the change in approaches to undergraduate medical education, with the development of problem based learning and the development of lifelong learning for practitioners.[2] The late 1990s and early 21st century saw the publication of a whole raft of books,[3–5] workbooks[6] and articles in peer-reviewed journals,[7–11] as well as workshops and seminars promoting evidence based healthcare.

Healthcare workers want to provide care to their patients which is likely to have a positive impact on their health outcome – to provide healthcare that is appropriate for the patient's condition, that is acceptable to the patient and that is known to be cost-effective. Where do they get the evidence to put this into their daily practice?

No busy clinician has the time to read the dozens of journal articles that are published every week in their field. The development of local and national guidelines has given clinicians information for planning and delivering health-care. In 1994, a randomised controlled trial in East London testing the effect of local asthma and diabetes guidelines' dissemination to non-training practices was completed.[12] The trial served as a model for a subsequent guidelines programme, was widely cited and was one of the first health services research papers abstracted in the journal *Evidence-based Medicine*. But, as Griffiths and Feder later stated, many of the earlier guidelines were consensus rather than evidence based.[13]

Organisations such as the Centre for Dissemination and Reviews at York University and the Cochrane Collaboration provide evidence based materials which can be easily digested. However, it is still up to the individual clinician, healthcare planner or manager to choose whether or not to read and to act on these.

The development of national standards

In April 1998 the concept of National Service Frameworks (NSFs) was launched to provide a structured basis on which to improve health and reduce inequalities. The remit of each NSF is shown in Box 10.1.

Box 10.1: National Service Frameworks

- Set national standards and define service models for a defined service or care group.
- Put in place strategies to support implementation.
- Establish performance milestones against which progress with an agreed timescale will be measured.
- Form one of a range of measures to raise quality and decrease variation in service.

It is expected that one NSF will be published each year and that all healthcare providers will work towards the standards they contain. Much of the challenge of implementation rests with primary care. It is recognised that implementing this agenda at a time of considerable change is a huge task for all primary care organisations and one that will require fundamental changes at both practice and primary care trust (PCT) level. Several NSFs have already been published and a work programme for the development and dissemination of others is in place. The Diabetes Services Delivery Strategy was published in 2002. The Renal NSF is next, followed by the Children's NSF and then the Long-Term Conditions NSF.

Box 10.2: NSFs to date

- Mental Health   September 1999
- Coronary Heart Disease   March 2000
- The Cancer Plan   September 2000
- Older People   March 2001
- Diabetes Services (Standards)   December 2001

Health professionals, service users and carers, health service managers, partner agencies and other advocates are represented on an external reference group for each NSF.

The initial development of NSFs was followed, in 1999, by the establishment of the National Institute for Clinical Excellence (NICE) as a special health authority for England and Wales. NICE provides a focus for clear, consistent guidelines for clinicians about which treatments work best for particular groups of patients. The definitions of the type/level of evidence used in the NICE guidelines originate from the US Agency for Health Care Policy and Research published in 1992. This ranges from level Ia evidence from meta-analysis of randomised controlled trials to level IV evidence from expert committee reports or opinions and/or clinical experience of respected authorities. The derivation and grading of recommendations is then based on a publication by Eccles *et al.*[14]

Continuing professional development is crucial to ensure that clinicians and others involved in the delivery and management of healthcare are able to understand and practise evidence based healthcare. Lifelong learning allows NHS staff to identify training needs across professional boundaries.

The Department of Health (DoH) has produced or commissioned a number of tools to assist practitioners to find and implement evidence. The *Information for Health* strategy has played a large part in bringing evidence to the desk and desktop of the GP, nurse, manager and other primary care professionals, through the development of the NHSnet and advances in the use of clinical computers.[15]

Another useful tool from the DoH is the resource pack *National Service Frameworks: a practical aid to implementation in primary care.*[16] This pack has been distributed to all GP practices, NSF and clinical governance leads, nurses working in primary and community care, allied health professionals, information technology leads and practice managers. It is therefore designed to be of benefit to both PCTs and individual practices in taking forward the NSF agenda. It is recognised that the information may be best used as an interprofessional framework or tool for development and can be linked to the practice development plan. It is also acknowledged that there are certain generic requirements that are probably common to all of the NSFs. These areas include organisational issues and ways of working that underpin the integration of clinical activity based around the needs of patients. The pack has 11 booklets, which are listed in Box 10.3.

Box 10.3: NSFs: a practical aid to implementation in primary care

- Introduction.
- Developing the information systems.
- Health improvement and prevention.
- Addressing inequalities – reaching the hard-to-reach groups.
- Screening/case finding.
- Chronic disease management and self-care.
- Referrals.
- Organisational development.
- Best practice.
- Partnership working.
- Funding streams.

Each booklet contains a short section on the national contribution, which is followed with suggestions about what the practice and the PCT can do to implement the evidence on that particular aspect. The booklets also contain background information, resources for further information and are illustrated with case studies from around the country.

The National electronic Library for Health

Why do we need a National electronic Library for Health (NeLH)?

In relation to the professional knowledge base, NHS professionals cannot possibly retain in their heads all current and emerging knowledge about the work they do.[15]

The public and NHS staff will be able to access information on local care services and how best to use them through nhs.uk and evidence based information and clinical guidelines through the National electronic Library for Health.[17]

The NeLH provides a useful first stop for those seeking to put clinical evidence into everyday practice. The site provides links to NICE and other guidelines, to *Clinical Evidence*, the Cochrane Library, Medline/Pubmed and evidence based journals such as *Bandolier*. Doctors and nurses are clearly not the only people with access to clinical evidence. Patients often arrive in the consulting room with information downloaded from the Internet or having read reports of clinical research that have been published in the national press. The NeLH provides information and critical appraisal of the research behind the stories through 'Hitting the Headlines'. Researchers from the NHS Centre for Reviews and Dissemination based at the University of York produce a one- or two-page appraisal (*see* Box 10.4).

Box 10.4: 'Hitting the Headlines': appraisal

- Where does the evidence come from?
- What were the authors' objectives?
- What was the nature of the evidence?
- What interventions were examined in the research?
- What were the findings?
- What were the authors' conclusions?
- How reliable are the conclusions?
- Is there information about any related systematic review?
- Of the references and resources, which included information for patients?

NeLH also provides links to training materials, e.g. the Cochrane Library by Kate Light, and NeLH for practice managers and NeLH for practice nurses. These contain exercises that can be used for self-tuition or for training in groups.

There is also a specific primary care section of the NeLH (www.nelh-pc.nhs.uk) authored and maintained by the Primary Care Informatics Group at St George's Hospital Medical School (www.gpinformatics.org). It is popular with primary care and has over 700 000 hits per month and rising. It is focused on 'information-centred' knowledge management in the consulting room, concentrating on the dissemination of existing knowledge.[11] It is particularly used at the end of the morning and throughout the afternoon.

Box 10.5: NeLH-PC technical features

- Signposts to key papers and modernisation agenda – produced daily.
- Personalisation – 'My NeLH-PC'.
- Searchable electronic index – metadata.
- Special EBM search engine – three-tier searching: Guidelines, Summary of EBM, Medline clinical queries.
- Flat hierarchical structure – moving from Graphical User Interface (GUI) to flexible database-driven interface.
- Appropriate re-authoring.

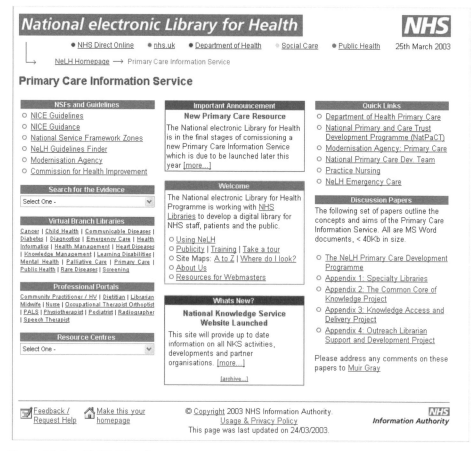

Figure 10.1: NeLH-PC web pages.

Primary Care Information Service (PRIMIS)

PRIMIS is a Department of Health-funded project to support improvements in data quality in primary care. It aims to help primary care organisations to improve patient care through the effective use of the clinical computer system. PRIMIS works with locally funded facilitators, to whom it provides training and support, to provide practices and PCTs with:

- guidance on making best use of clinical systems
- training and support to practice teams
- assistance with analyses of data quality
- feedback and interpretation of the results of the data quality analysis.

An example of how PRIMIS can support the implementation strategies at a PCT level is given below.

Putting clinical evidence into daily practice: collaboration in east London

We would like to illustrate this section of the chapter with a description of the work of the Clinical Effectiveness Group (CEG), based in the academic Department of General Practice and Primary Care at Queen Mary University of London. The CEG has supported national initiatives around the NSFs and NHS modernisation, prioritising chronic disease management and an integrated approach to the implementation of evidence based primary care.

The CEG has established good working relationships with the three local PCTs – City and Hackney, Newham and Tower Hamlets – with each PCT represented on the CEG steering group.

One of the recommendations of the 'Developing the Information Systems' section of *National Service Frameworks: a practical aid to implementation in primary care*[16] is the development of a common data set. CEG has played a key role in this development in east London, and in 2002, 86 per cent of east London practices were contributing electronically to this data set for chronic disease management. The data set includes an electronic coronary heart disease (CHD) register comprising 12 000 people and high quality data on their care.

The CEG developed in 1998 from two local initiatives which had been established in the 1980s by doctors and nurses from local general practices: the Healthy Eastenders Project, which focused on prevention of coronary heart disease, smoking-related cancer, cervical and breast cancer; and the East London

Guidelines Project, which developed chronic disease management and other guidelines appropriate for the local population. Both projects employed facilitators to work with local practices and incorporated clinical audit in their activity. The CEG further developed the audit and became a pilot site for the Collection of Health Data from General Practice (CHDGP), the predecessor of PRIMIS.

Box 10.6: Continuing professional development (CPD) in the clinical environment

- Uses related to the practice clinical system: patient registration, registration links, medical history, consultations, templates/protocols, referrals, prescribing, clinical links, audit and searching, knowledge systems such as PRODIGY.
- Uses related to standard business software: word processing, spreadsheets, email, Internet, intranets.
- Other clinical uses: NHSnet (information, electronic textbooks, distance learning, email).

Sharing Quality in Data (SQUID), the CEG audit, is part of the PRIMIS data collection network. Practices can sign up to audit and facilitation on coronary heart disease (*see* Figure 10.2), asthma, long-term mental illness and depression. These are supported by templates for the clinical computer system and data are extracted either electronically through the MIQUEST interpreter or by an audit of the paper records if this is not possible.

Box 10.7: Sharing Quality in Data

Pan east London project facilitating improved quality and use of primary care clinical information to:

- develop and promote use of computerised disease registers
- establish common data sets
- collect and collate data from those registers using MIQUEST
- feed back results to practices
- support practices in implementing change
- participate in NHS Information Authority national PRIMIS programme.

Box 10.8: What is MIQUEST?

- Morbidity Information Query Export Syntax.
- Writes searches in health query language (HQL).
- Searches on: Read codes, *British National Formulary* headings and system-generated codes.
- Cannot extract patient-identifiable data.
- Requires each clinical system to have an interpreter.
- This is a requirement for accreditation (RFA 99) for clinical system vendors.

CEG facilitators provide in-practice education across both clinical governance and clinical guidelines. This is complemented by postgraduate meetings in local centres, work with small practices and the nurse forum meetings.

In 2001, CEG worked with 123 practices in east London (82 per cent of all practices) on the development of registers for diabetes. Electronic diabetes audits were conducted in 91, while manual audits were provided by 32 practices (*see* Table 10.1).

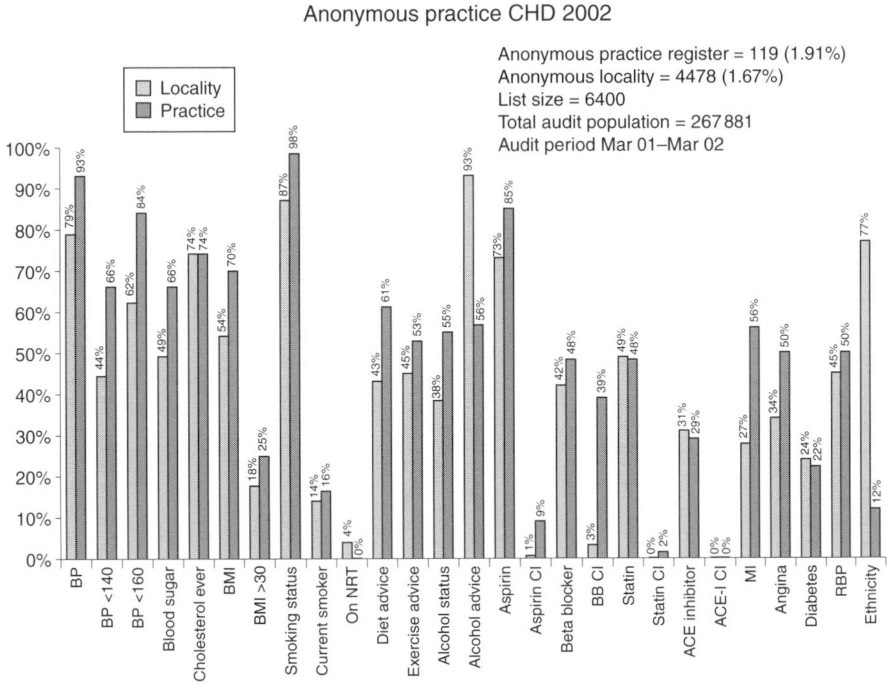

Figure 10.2: Anonymised practice CHD data in 2002.

Table 10.1: CEG audit results for diabetes in Tower Hamlets practices for 2001

Audit features	2000	2001
No. of participating practices	18	34
Diabetes population	2739	5623
Prevalence	2.4%	3.1%
Type 1 or	12.6%	10%
Type 2 diabetes	60%	62%
Type not recorded	27.4%	28%
Urine test for protein recorded	44%	37%
BMI recorded	54%	57%
Feet: full examination recorded	26%	25%
Eyes: full examination recorded	33%	22%
Blood pressure recorded	77%	74%
Systolic control <140 mmHg	54%	47%
HbA1c or fructosamine measured	56%	55%
HbA1c <8%		24%
Creatinine measured	45%	51%
Cholesterol measured	42%	47%
Smoking history ever recorded	90%	90%
Current smoker	23%	12%
Smoking advice to current smokers recorded	27%	27%
Dietary advice given		31%
Absolute 10-year CHD risk assessed		16%
Place of annual review: GP		11%
Hospital		42%

Data are presented electronically, in paper format and in practice based education meetings by CEG facilitators. Practices receive data for their own patients with comparative data showing change over time within their own practice. Receiving data for their locality and for the total of the three localities enables comparison with other practices. This information is most useful if practices are able to see beyond the data and use it to review the case given to individual patients.

In addition to its education and facilitation programme, the CEG currently supports data extraction, analysis and administration of those parts of the General Medical Services (GMS) contract linked to chronic disease management, i.e. health promotion, chronic disease management (CDM) and sustained quality payments. The PCT-led initiatives, i.e. CHD and diabetes incentive schemes, are also supported in a similar way. This occurs across the three PCT areas of east London and is undertaken in collaboration with the clinical governance, primary care development and finance departments of those PCTs. The CEG has also agreed to support monitoring of the Personal Medical Services (PMS) contract for one of the PCTs from April 2003.

The new GP contract introduces new dimensions to monitoring within primary care.[18] Over time, all PCTs will develop the capabilities to undertake the level of standard setting and monitoring required by the new quality markers. However, until robust systems are in place we believe that the CEG has a role in supporting PCTs in delivering the information required as follows:

1 **Accurate disease registers** are the cornerstone of effective and high quality CDM. As described above, the CEG now uses predicted prevalence of chronic disease (linked to individual practice demographic profiles) to identify those practices that are under-diagnosing patients. Practice data quality searches (PDQs) which compare actual recording of diagnosis with the monitoring codes for that specific condition can also be utilised. However, this method is open to considerable clinical interpretation with discrepancies occurring naturally within the data. We can provide a combination of analysis on each practice's disease registers across a range of conditions.

2 **Template designs** using agreed quality indicators are required to promote consistent recording of data. The CEG has proven experience in developing templates, liaising with national organisations and utilising local expert opinion to produce agreed quality indicator sets. We can develop these templates so that there is consistency and comparability across the new strategic health authority. A systematic programme of template loading (including clearing of existing templates) is required in conjunction with an educational programme.

3 **New organisational criteria** are required by the contract, including 'exception reporting' for those patients who are considered appropriate for excluding. Searches on such criteria can be developed and run on an annual basis as required by the PCTs. At present the national data extraction PRIMIS centre does not adapt its searches for individual PCTs; their comparable audits (CAS) are run to a set timetable on a regular annual basis.

4 **Training** of primary care and all attached staff is essential to the success of improving data quality and the implementation of the contract. The CEG can support locality PCT facilitators, based either at the CEG or the PCTs, in facilitation of: improving accuracy of disease registers, loading templates and then using them during the clinical consultation, feedback of clinical audits and promoting evidence based care. The CEG has recently met with the east London PCT's IM&T managers and trainers to discuss how to support improved data quality in practices. PRIMIS training can be made available to the PCT trainers and regular PDQ searches can also be run by PRIMIS. Clinical searches can be retained locally, feeding into the PRIMIS CAS service as and when their timetable allows, for national comparisons.

5 **Contract monitoring** – a 'high trust reporting' programme is outlined in the GP contract. Practices will be required to submit or be available for audit verification by the PCTs. The CEG currently manages to engage 90% of east London practices and 94% of the population in a voluntary audit programme including the analysis. The analysis is reported back both to the PCTs via reports and the individual practices via a practice based multidisciplinary educational programme.

It is expected that the most reliable and effective way to monitor the GP contract will be through developments within the main clinical system suppliers. Given that the new contract will base much of its remuneration on the provision of good data, EMIS and other suppliers will be responsible for producing standard searches built into their software that will provide practices with the information that they can supply to the PCTs in support of their claims. Current indications would suggest that a system similar to that used to provide results for cervical cytology and immunisations will be adopted.

Putting evidence into daily practice: in general practice

Audit is often seen as a number-crunching exercise with little relation to the practice or individual patient. The scenario described below illustrates how this need not be the case. One morning, by chance, very few patients attended the diabetes clinic to see the GP or practice nurse. The GP decided to use the protected time for the clinic to carry out an audit of his patients with diabetes. The audit and the meaning behind the numbers is given in the case study below.

Case study: Care of patients with diabetes
Using the practice clinical system, a GP in east London conducted an audit of patients registered with him who had diabetes – 62 patients. The audit looked at the number of patients seen in the last year for a review of their diabetes and who had an HbA1c recorded. He also audited the HbA1c as a measure of good control.

There were 62 diabetic patients, of whom two had type 1 diabetes.

Six patients had not had their HbA1c checked within the past year.
Two of these were middle-aged men who were known to be staying for quite long periods in Bangladesh. One man had recently been seen in the diabetic clinic but he had deliberately avoided having any blood tests. Another had been seen within the past two months to discuss her diabetic control, and had agreed to come for blood tests, but had not done so. Two others had not

been seen for quite some time – one man who had not been back in contact with the surgery after an initial diagnosis of diabetes the previous year, and another man who had failed to respond to written appointment requests both from our clinic and the hospital diabetes clinic.

Seven people had an HbA1c above 11% (fructosamine >600).

One of these was a late adolescent with type 1 diabetes, whose diabetes has been very difficult to control for several years – and whose capacity to control it has in fact been markedly improved in the past year or so, with a decrease in hospital admissions in ketoacidosis.

Of those with type 2 diabetes, one had had fairly recent onset of disease and clearly needs more treatment which has now been started – his diabetes may have been made worse by olanzapine recently. Of those who had not had their treatment increased, there was a significant contribution to the problems of their management from language problems and related transcultural gulfs of comprehension and communication about our different understandings of diabetes. One of the eight, newly diagnosed, had already clearly responded well to an increase in her treatment.

Ten people had an HbA1c above 9%, below 11% (fructosamine >550).

All ten had type 2 diabetes. One was a severely disabled elderly man with a long-term mental illness and extrapyramidal movement disorder who is looked after by relatives but takes his treatment irregularly. Another had recently defaulted from a hospital referral, is a heavy smoker with arterial disease and BMI above 30, taking insulin – so advised resume metformin. Another was a new patient on diet alone, so drug treatment started. Another three had had their oral treatment increased. One elderly patient on insulin attends the hospital diabetic clinic; another, on rosiglitazone and glibenclamide who cannot tolerate metformin but has arterial disease, has been referred back to the clinic having previously defaulted. Another on maximal doses of gliclazide and metformin had had diet advice reiterated. Another relatively new diabetic seems to need higher doses but this was deferred because of travel abroad.

Nine people had an HbA1c above 8%, below 9% (fructosamine >500).

Of these type 2 diabetics, three were arteriopaths whose treatment with oral hypoglycaemics had been increased at their last review. Two others without arterial disease had also had treatment increases. One person who had rather reluctantly been persuaded to start oral treatment a year ago was on gliclazide 80 mg bd. Another who was on insulin, metformin and orlistat had defaulted hospital follow-up and was not really taking much metformin. Another on metformin 1700 mg daily had agreed to try to lose more weight by diet and exercise. In one case needing better treatment there seemed to be confusion about treatment, associated with language and trans-cultural difficulties of care.

Seven people had HbA1c above 7%, below 8% (fructosamine >450).

One was a type 1 diabetic with an extremely irregular lifestyle, who titrated short-acting insulin doses against diet and exercise in a very dynamic self-management regime.

Of the six type 2 diabetics, three had had appropriate increases in their drug regimes at review. One was a relatively new diabetic on diet who did not want to start drugs. Two others on gliclazide had had advice about diet.

Actions taken after this review of diabetic control.

It was decided to focus on those who had not had their HbA1c measured at all but who were in the country, using letters and telephone calls. Also to try to recheck HbA1cs that are above 8% every six months or sooner, to try to get them below that level, particularly focusing, using advocates where possible, on those where difficulties of understanding of diabetes seemed to be a key factor. It was hoped that with these efforts, the 43% incidence of HbA1c greater than 8% – that is, of very poor control – could perhaps be reduced to 20%.

As this audit shows, there are a number of factors which can affect patient out-come. These include practice and patient factors. How patients are informed that they have a condition such as diabetes, and their response to this, impacts on their management and outcome. If patients do not attend for blood tests or annual review or choose to stay away from the practice completely, this can affect their outcome.

The case study also raises issues of access to services and the need to make sure that services are culturally sensitive. The practice is fortunate to work with Sylheti/Bengali and Chinese/Vietnamese-speaking health advocates who have regular sessions in the practice. The practice can also book advocates for Somali, Albanian and French-speaking patients. The health advocates contact patients who are booked into the diabetes clinic before their appointment time to check that they will be coming and to encourage those having doubts. The advocates also contact patients who do not attend to discuss their reasons and to try to encourage them to rebook their appointment.

Co-morbidity is another important factor. The patients with long-standing mental health problems also had poor control of their diabetes. Behind the audit figures there are complex stories of human lives. In putting clinical evidence into everyday practice, the GP, practice nurse and health advocate have to acknowledge those stories and, for each individual patient, try to work out the most appropriate way of working with them to accept and manage their diabetes.

This illustrates many of the points made earlier.[16] The booklet *Addressing Inequalities – reaching the hard-to-reach groups* acknowledges the significantly different health outcomes for men and women. Male life expectancy is still lower than that for women and the gap is wider for men from less affluent backgrounds. Contributory factors include differences in frequency of access to health services and that men are more likely to be susceptible to the wider determinants of ill health such as poverty and unemployment.

Practices are encouraged to work with the PCT to ensure comprehensive healthcare provision is available to marginalised groups such as refugees and asylum seekers, and to ensure access to health advocates.

Conclusions

Most published accounts of successful implementation of evidence based practice are presented as teamwork successes. On occasion the 'hard liners' for the evidence based agenda discover that the environment of NHS service delivery, with an emphasis on using available data and information systems, can be unpredictable.[19] The idea of multidisciplinary practice education is gaining momentum and is being recognised as the way forward in initiating and sustaining positive changes within an organisation.[20]

References

1 Department of Health (1998) *A First Class Service: quality in the new NHS.* HMSO, London.

2 General Medical Council (2002) *Tomorrow's Doctors. Recommendations on undergraduate medical education.* General Medical Council, London.

3 Sackett DL, Richardson SR, Rosenberg W *et al.* (1997) *Evidence-based Medicine: how to practise and teach EBM.* Churchill Livingstone, London.

4 Muir Gray JA (1997) *Evidence-based Healthcare: how to make health policy and management decisions.* Churchill Livingstone, London.

5 Ridsdale L (ed.) (1998) *Evidence-based Medicine in Primary Care.* Churchill Livingstone, London.

6 Carter YH and Falshaw M (eds) (1998) *Evidence-based Primary Care: an open learning programme.* Radcliffe Medical Press, Oxford.

7 Haines A and Donald A (1998) Getting research findings into practice. Making better use of research findings. *BMJ.* **317:** 72–5.

8 Sheldon TA, Guyatt GH and Haines A (1998) Getting research findings into practice. When to act on the evidence. *BMJ.* **317:** 39–42.

9   Greenhalgh T (1997) *How to Read a Paper: the basics of evidence-based medicine*. British Medical Journal Publishing Group, London.

10 McColl A, Smith H, White P *et al.* (1998) General practitioners' perceptions of the route to evidence-based medicine: a questionnaire survey. *BMJ.* **316**: 361–5.

11 Sackett DL, Rosenberg WM, Muir Gray JA *et al.* (1996) Evidence-based medicine: what it is and what it isn't. *BMJ.* **312**: 71–2.

12 Feder G, Griffiths C, Highton C *et al.* (1995) Do clinical guidelines introduced with practice-based education improve care of asthmatic and diabetic patients? *BMJ.* **311**: 473–8.

13 Griffiths C and Feder G (1998) Can we improve our management of acute asthma? An approach to using clinical guidelines. In: L Ridsdale (ed.) *Evidence-based Medicine in Primary Care*. Churchill Livingstone, London.

14 Eccles M, Freemantle N and Mason J (1998) North of England evidence based guideline development project: guideline for angiotensin converting enzyme inhibitors in primary care management of adults with symptomatic heart failure. *BMJ.* **316**: 1369–75.

15 National Health Service Executive (1998) *Information for Health. An information strategy for the modern NHS 1998–2005. A national strategy for local implementation*. Department of Health, HMSO, London.

16 Department of Health (2002) *National Service Frameworks: a practical aid to implementation in primary care*. HMSO, London.

17 Department of Health (2000) *The NHS Plan – a plan for investment, a plan for reform*. HMSO, London.

18 General Practitioners Committee (2002) *Your Contract, Your Future*. British Medical Association, London.

19 Lipman T and Price D (2000) Decision making, evidence, audit, and education: case study of antibiotic prescribing in general practice. *BMJ.* **320**: 1114–18.

20 Greenhalgh T (2000) Commentary: what can we learn from narratives of implementing evidence. *BMJ.* **320**: 1118–19.

CHAPTER 11

Work based learning and overseas development

Neil Jackson, Pamela Jackson, Patrick MacCarthy and Deirdre MacCarthy

And by experience it is known to me that there are two kinds of counsel: that which procedeth from the tongue and that which proceedeth from the heart. I turned my ear to that which procedeth from the tongue: but to the counsel of the heart, which I heard, I gave a place in the treasury of my soul.

(Emperor Tamerlane, 1336–1405)

Introduction

In this chapter the authors will recount their activities as visiting primary care educationalists in supporting the development of in-service training programmes for general practitioners and primary healthcare services in the republics of Georgia and Uzbekistan. We gratefully acknowledge the opportunity given to us to support these development programmes through the close collaboration of various organisations including: the World Bank; the Department for International Development (DfID); Health and Life Sciences Partnership (HLSP Ltd); the London Deanery (formerly the North Thames East Deanery); and the respective ministries of health for Georgia and Uzbekistan.

We are also indebted to the Georgian and Uzbek doctors participating in the in-service training programmes for their commitment, enthusiasm and continuing friendship.

Historical background

Until the late 1980s the USSR rivalled the USA as a military and political superpower. It is now a matter of history that with the catalyst of events in Russia and

East Germany, the USSR broke up in the early 1990s and this resulted in many of the former republics of that bloc becoming independent countries. Georgia and Uzbekistan were two such 'new' countries that found themselves largely detached from the centralised control and economic security blanket that had cocooned them for the previous 70 years.

Independence is usually perceived as an opportunity for national advancement, but when it comes about unexpectedly it can also be a time of economic, political and social destabilisation.

Georgia was afflicted with a civil war and an almost non-existent economy. Uzbekistan had very strong political control but suffered wage reductions, rampant inflation and major GDP decline.

Inevitably this period of economic dysfunction has had ramifications for the health systems of these countries. Until the break-up of the USSR, healthcare policy throughout the republics was controlled from Moscow and administered by the relevant local ministries. As in the UK, care was free at the point of contact. Funding was from specified budget allowances that were decided centrally. With the financial difficulties faced by both countries, resource allocation to healthcare was compromised. In 1998 Georgia spent 0.6% of GDP on healthcare, and Uzbekistan spent 2.9% in 1999. This compares with 7.1% for the UK and a CEE (Central and Eastern Europe) average of 5.7% in 1998.[1]

Under the 'old' system the emphasis on health delivery was through secondary rather than primary care. There were large numbers of hospital based doctors and many hospital beds (ten times the number of beds per person available in the UK). Primary care in the form of family medicine with general practitioners and primary care nurses did not exist. Instead care was partly supplied in urban settings by a system of polyclinics. These were centrally sited, state-run community clinics, each caring for tens of thousands of patients. Many doctors were employed but on low incomes. Separate clinics with their own staff laboratory and X-ray facilities existed for adults, children and women's (antenatal and gynaecological) healthcare. Preventive programmes such as immunisation and cervical screening were conducted from these. Medical care within the polyclinic system was doctor-dominant with little opportunity for nurse input. Care was divided into many specialities within the polyclinic but expertise was not of a level that would be associated with a speciality in the UK. Doctors did not appear to have the encouragement or opportunity to gain experience outside their own confined field of work.

The old, inefficient model of healthcare delivery was clearly not going to be sustainable in the economic world to which the new republics were now being exposed. Both Georgia and Uzbekistan looked to develop a programme of re-training of doctors to become primary care physicians who would offer a more holistic approach to their populations, similar to that of GPs in the UK. The intention was that this would be a better use of human resources and a change in emphasis from secondary care prioritisation. Primary care was perceived as the most appropriate mechanism for healthcare to be supplied to countries where spending per head could be as little as $10/year compared to over $1500/year in western Europe.

It was in this context that a number of educational visits to Georgia and Uzbekistan were undertaken by the authors on behalf of the DfID with the purpose of assisting in the retraining of physicians to become trainers for future primary care workers in these countries.

The purpose of educational intervention in the development of overseas primary care systems

There are many significant principles which will underpin the future development of an overseas primary care health system. Some of these principles were set out in our own government's White Paper on the new NHS published in 1997[2] and in an overseas development context the following are worthy of consideration:

- a national service of healthcare
- an emphasis on appropriate responsibility at all levels in the developing healthcare system
- a partnership approach by the key stakeholders (i.e. government, organisational, team and professional)
- an efficient system of healthcare with quality of care for all patients.

The concept of quality should embrace both the patients' experience of healthcare and appropriate clinical outcomes. Quality in a developing healthcare system can only be promoted by a 'three systems approach,[3] i.e. service delivery and development, supported and informed by education and training, and research and development.

It follows that any educational intervention in an overseas context should be designed to provide maximum benefit to the developing primary healthcare system by supporting its workforce of healthcare professionals, both medical and non-medical. This recognises the need to establish highly skilled and integrated multidisciplinary teams of healthcare professionals who must work and learn together to deliver the future primary care agenda. The educational intervention must also address the issues of staff recruitment and retention and promote teamworking across organisational boundaries as well as professional boundaries. It is also important to ensure that primary care staff are equipped with the individual skills they need to work in the complexity of the developing healthcare system itself.

Over the past few years we have seen an increasing movement towards WBL in primary care in our own NHS. This is in keeping with Foster's definition of WBL being based on:

- the involvement of working teams in joint learning
- the relationship between learning and performance.[4]

The relationship between learning and performance in particular deserves recognition in any developing primary healthcare system at government, healthcare system, organisational, team and professional levels.

Drawing on their own experiences of working in the NHS, the authors utilised a work based learning approach while working as a multidisciplinary team of educationalists in the developing primary care systems in Uzbekistan and Georgia. One crucial objective of the educational intervention itself was to highlight many of the concepts and issues described above.

Can WBL benefit developing primary care systems?

It would be encouraging to think that WBL can be beneficial not only to developing primary care systems but also to other systems of healthcare that are in a state of evolution. By utilising the education and learning opportunities that occur in the workplace and trying to evaluate them under the three headings of for, at and from work, it may be possible through education and development for the whole workplace to improve many aspects of healthcare.

WBL can be used to promote higher standards of patient care by looking primarily at the requirements of patients, as it is their problems that are central to the considerations of any new or developing service. It could also encourage all professional groups to seek to provide the correct patient pathways through the development of joint learning and the improvement of interprofessional relationships. Not only is it beneficial to improve communications between professionals at all levels, but it is also important to redefine roles to maximise efficiency in all aspects of care distribution. This appears to be of particular importance in developing primary care systems where counterproductive hierarchical structures are so ingrained and especially in the presence of very restricted funding which seems to afflict new systems.

From a primary care workforce perspective WBL presents an opportunity for healthcare professionals at the 'coal face' to precipitate positive change in the system in which they work by a 'bottom up' approach. This is the reverse of the recognised approach of change being instigated from above for political and management reasons and being promoted downwards to a compliant and accepting workforce. Thus ethical issues such as resource allocation within developing primary care systems may be subject to a broader scrutiny that should be beneficial to the majority of patients.

While continuing to be perceived as a threat by many, appraisal and competence assessment are realities of modern healthcare practice. WBL may well be one of a number of tools to look at patient care from different perspectives and may be used to evaluate different levels of input from all members of the primary care team. It is hoped that in the WBL context, service development and educational benefit might be seen as a joint goal.

Case scenarios to illustrate work based learning in a developing primary care system

The authors used a variety of teaching methods during several trips to Tashkent (Republic of Uzbekistan) and Tbilisi (Republic of Georgia). These included various clinical case scenarios, based on previous actual consultations in general practice or a community setting in the United Kingdom. Each case scenario illustrated various aspects of work based learning, i.e. learning for work, learning at work and learning from work. The case scenarios were used in large- or small-group work with trainee family physicians.

Case scenario 11.1
A 30-year-old mother of two children aged two and five months presents to a family planning nurse in a community based family planning clinic for contraceptive advice. She has suffered a deep vein thrombosis in the past and feels her family is now complete.

This case scenario illustrates the following aspects of work based learning.

Learning for work
- Knowledge base/awareness of the range of methods of contraception.
- Awareness of side effects/contraindications of each method of contraception.
- Risks of unwanted pregnancy/efficacy of each method of contraception.

Learning at work
- The importance of good record-keeping and the use of patient records as a tool for quality patient care.
- Learning from patients by a patient-centred approach (addressing the patients' ideas, concerns and expectations).
- The various aspects of patient management, e.g. what investigations are appropriate in this consultation?

Learning from work
- Shared learning between family planning doctors and nurses in respect of their professional roles in patient management.
- Managing risk in a primary care setting.
- Developing management protocols for family planning.

Case scenario 11.2
A male patient aged 18 presents to a general practitioner with a sore throat of three days' duration and he requests a prescription for antibiotics.
   This case scenario illustrates the following aspects of work based learning.

Learning for work
- Background knowledge of the likely causes of sore throats.
- The evidence base for the use of antibiotics.
- Possible side effects of antibiotics.

Learning at work
- Practice audit meetings to review antibiotic prescribing.
- Checking the appropriate dosage of specific antibiotics as necessary.
- Assessing the patient's ability to cope with minor illness.

Learning from work
- Teaching trainee general practitioners about the appropriate use of antibiotic prescribing.
- Reviewing the cost of antibiotic prescribing in primary care.
- The pros and cons of nurse prescribing/developing nurse prescribing protocols.

Case scenario 11.3
An eight-year-old boy presents to the practice nurse with a history of a persistent night cough and increasing shortness of breath on exercise.

Learning for work
- Knowledge of the anatomy, physiology and pathology of obstructive airways disease.
- Awareness of national evidence based guidelines.
- Education in methods of diagnosing asthma/treatment options.
- Regular updating by resourcing journals, Internet, etc.

Learning at work
- Development of accurate history-taking skills and the use of a systematic approach.

- Utilisation of practice guidelines and protocols.
- The use of patient care plans thus ensuring safe and consistent practice.

Learning from work
- The value of patient/parent education in both the disease and treatment in order to promote medication compliance.
- Case review with colleagues.
- Cohort asthma therapy review.
- The importance of audit as a learning tool for the primary healthcare team.

Case scenario 11.4
A woman in her twenties presents to a general practitioner with abdominal pain.

Learning for work
- Updating knowledge of anatomy, physiology and pathology.
- Importance of an organised and systematic approach.
- Differential diagnoses to cover presenting problem.
- Prioritisation of diagnostic possibilities.
- Confirmation of adequacy of clinical examination skills.

Learning at work
- Ethical considerations, e.g. consent and confidentiality.
- Rapport with patient.
- Appreciation of cultural and social setting.
- History-taking skills.
- Examination skills/use of chaperones.
- Reaching provisional diagnoses.
- Appropriate confirmatory investigations.
- Taking responsibility and planning disposal.
- Giving uncertain diagnoses or bad news.
- Referral versus temporisation: concept of risk minimisation.
- Immediate requirements, e.g. analgesia.
- Importance of good record-keeping.

Learning from work
- Opportunity for case discussion.
- Did we get it right? Diagnostic/management review.
- Looking at deficiencies and planning accordingly.
- Audit.
- Consideration of development of protocols and use of flow charts.

The trainee perspective

During their consultancy visits to both Georgia and Uzbekistan the authors noted the ease with which trainee general practitioners identified with the WBL model. In Georgia, for example, the first eight GPs to be trained in the country were set the task of undertaking individual audit projects as a part of the training programme.

> **Vignette 11.1**
> One trainee GP used her previous experience of working in the Georgian healthcare system as a basis for reflection and change. Her project involved undertaking an audit of hypertension in a polyclinic in the light of modern thinking and the evidence base for the management of hypertension, with account taken of the restraints of the limited availability of antihypertensive drugs, scarcity of resources, etc., within the country.

Similar projects completed by the other trainee GPs were instrumental in introducing models of good practice into the developing Georgian healthcare system.

> **Vignette 11.2**
> While working in Uzbekistan, trainee general practitioners were encouraged to present patients for case discussion as a means of highlighting WBL and to enhance their presentation skills.
> A female patient in her mid-forties was presented to the visiting primary care consultants and the trainee group by an Uzbek trainee GP with a specialist interest in neurology. The patient had previously been investigated by various specialists for a bilateral tremor affecting her hands and arms. The differential diagnosis and management of the patient was considered by the group and the patient was encouraged to participate in the discussion. It was concluded that the probable diagnosis was that of benign familial tremor.

In WBL terms this case illustrated the importance of learning from patients in the workplace and in particular the physical, psychological and social impact of illness or disability in a primary care setting and looking at the patient's agenda and concerns.

WBL in developing healthcare systems: the future

An important issue to consider in establishing a WBL approach in a developing primary healthcare system is the effectiveness of learning for both healthcare teams and individual professionals.

The role of educational assessment through formative and summative feedback therefore becomes crucial. Linking assessment to learning will enhance professional and team performance by enabling identified educational needs to be met while recognising that individual and team performance is multi-dimensional. A system of assessment will also facilitate self-directed learning via a broad spectrum of both formal and informal educational opportunities and resources.

The principles and purpose of assessment will be addressed in more depth in the next chapter.

Although there are many other issues to consider for the future in relation to the WBL model in a developing primary care healthcare system, the question of who needs to be involved in supporting this is paramount. A summary of the interested parties is given in Box 11.1.

Box 11.1: Who needs to be involved in supporting the development of WBL

- Healthcare professionals (doctors, nurses, other professions allied to medicine).
- Primary care service provider organisations/teams (GP practices/clinics, etc.).
- Professional colleges/associations.
- Governments/ministries of health.
- Professional regulatory bodies.
- Educators/CPD providers.
- Patients/society.

References

1 European Observatory on Health Care (2001) Systems *Health Care Systems in Transition – Uzbekistan.* WHO Regional Office for Europe, Copenhagen.

2 Secretary of State for Health (1997) *The New NHS.* HMSO, London.

3 Jackson N (1999) Quality in the new NHS – the role of education and training in general practice and primary care. *Ed Gen Pract.* **10**: 6–8.

4 Foster E (1996) *Comparable but Different: work-based learning for a learning society.* DfEE and University of Leeds, Leeds.

CHAPTER 12

Work based learning in primary care: where to next?

Neil Jackson and Jonathan Burton

What must be changed? What can be kept? How best can the latter be amplified?
(William Boyd and Edmund King[1])

Revisiting the definition of work based learning

In the earlier chapters of this book we used a definition of work based learning which acknowledged the impact of work experiences on individual learning. Many of these are relatively unstructured and reactive, although no less important for being so. Our definition also covered the deliberate learning activities of individuals and teams, often taking place away from work, but designed to change individual and team capacities in terms of patient care.

Change in capacity

The place of work, with its huge variety of opportunities for learning, has a special significance in lifelong learning. This starts with the apprenticeship experiences of new entrants to a profession, who learn on the job, by observation, absorption and practice. It goes on to the career-long learning of the individual professions, where change in capacity on many fronts has to take place alongside the duties of daily work. This change in capacity is less and less left to chance or individual motivation. The basic purpose of the quality agenda (as covered especially in Chapters 9 and 10) is that patient care should be safe, efficient and effective. This means that capacity has to be demonstrated and proved.

What is right and what is wrong?

Many practitioners will rightly feel that they (and the teams in which they work) have long practised the disciplines of self-improvement and that they therefore have little more to do to sustain a continuing level of good and self-renewing performance. Many will also feel that, in the pressurised world in which they work, there is little room for further change. Indeed, in this book (*see* Chapter 3) we have emphasised the importance of sustainable learning. One of the most important aspects of work based learning is that it is practical and at hand.

However, we have emphasised that WBL can go wrong. Individual poor performance (as described in Chapter 8) is usually associated with a poorly orga- nised workplace and a failure to expose oneself to the many opportunities for peer review and self-improvement that are offered with work based learning. There are many traps in WBL, which have been covered in Chapter 3. Collabora- tive learning can be ineffective if the learning is badly organised, or is based on false information or other forms of incompleteness. Opportunities for learning arise constantly at work, but may be regularly or systematically neglected.

What will happen?

There are already new movements in place which are going to ensure that WBL becomes more effective and systematic. For example, there are the arrange- ments for appraisal of GPs. Much of the evidence for appraisal will be based on what is going on or not going on at work. It is not hard to predict that over the next few years GPs will become more systematic in their approach to WBL in response to these new requirements. It is likely that practice contracts, which will be performance and outcome based, will form the basis of new pay arrange- ments in primary care. In this way, the voluntarism which is now attached to much of the quality agenda will disappear. Teams which can adjust to the new system will flourish. Teams that flourish will be teams that already work well across the professions. Interprofessional learning will become a mainstream activity. Patients, too, will have influence, being better informed and demand- ing better services. All this suggests that external and societal changes will drive the changes in WBL.

Should WBL be managed or will it just evolve?

Is the job of government or management to negotiate and plan the desirable changes in the NHS, to establish the parameters by which success will be mea- sured, to set up the structures that will measure this success and then to leave local teams to get on with things? Or is it also to manage the local teams, to assist them in their development as they attempt to achieve the set objectives? Is the creativity that underlies the success of individuals and teams to be valued as the prime driving force of change and renewal? Or should individuals and teams be helped (by various forms of assessment) to achieve what has been set out? To end this book, we now set out some of the ways in which WBL could be systematically assessed.

The principles and purpose of assessment as applied to WBL

The important link between WBL and assessment has already been highlighted in Chapter 11 with particular reference to ensuring that learning is effective for healthcare teams and professionals. The principles and purpose of assessment are now well established[2,3] and a broad range of methods of assessment are used extensively and systematically to determine clinical competence and performance in healthcare professionals. One example is the system of formative and summative assessment established in the GP registrar year of the general practice vocational training programme.

Competence may be defined as the possession of sufficient ability expressed in terms of knowledge, skills and attitudes, i.e. what you 'can do'. Performance on the other hand refers to what you 'actually do' in fulfilling or accomplishing the duties and tasks required of the individual healthcare professional.

Assessment has a critical part to play in any educational process. Wherever learning takes place, or it is intended that it should take place, it is entirely reasonable for the learner, the teacher (or tutor) and other interested parties or organisations to be curious about the learning process and its outcomes.

A variety of assessment methods can be applied in WBL in a formative sense to enhance clinical competence and performance. These include:

- confidence rating scales
- attitudinal questionnaires
- sitting in
- review of consultation record
- video analysis of consultations
- feedback from patients, colleagues and staff
- random case analysis
- problem case analysis
- preparation of teaching sessions
- MCQs
- EMQs

- MEQs
- OSCEs
- project and audit work
- practice exchange visits.

As WBL develops in the future, any link to assessment must be carefully considered, particularly in relation to issues of feasibility and the application of assessment methodology.

A more systematic approach to WBL

Chance cannot be removed entirely from learning. Nor can the definition of what should be learned be exactly delineated. In fact, there are disadvantages in trying to do so, so varied are the needs of patients – and therefore learning should be equally varied, flexible and responsive.

But clearly WBL will become more disciplined and structured. In some of this there will be no choice. Unavoidable external influences will impinge on primary care. These will be: appraisal, outcome-related practice contracts (which will encompass the quality agenda), the changing expectations of patients and greater ease of access to relevant information – especially through the medium of IT. Many of these areas have already been addressed in some detail in this book.

This should benefit both practitioners and patients. Practitioners will develop the habit of learning, on a daily basis, and in a sustainable but effective way. Primary care teams will make their practice based learning equally productive and to the point. Quicker access to information will make uncertainty or ignorance a matter which can be declared as readily as it can be resolved. These external influences, in turn, should reduce the use of bluff (Chapter 1, Chapter 7), misinformation (Chapter 3), bad organisation of care (Chapter 9) and blocking (Chapter 7), all of which affect the relationship between practitioners and patients.

Making WBL more effective

These unavoidable external influences will force up the general standards of performance but they will not identify or remedy the more subtle differences between individual practitioners or teams. One team may be doing fairly well (in its own view), but might have a lot to learn from how a neighbouring team organises care. Year on year of 'practising in a vacuum' can make individuals and teams unaware of what they might be achieving. In its worst aspect, this process is associated with dangerously poor performance (Chapter 8), but it affects everyone. Submitting oneself or one's team to the sort of review processes listed in the section on formative assessment (above) will be the best way of guaranteeing that unintended problems are not left unidentified.

References

1 Boyd W and King E (1964) *The History of Western Education.* A & C Black, London.

2 MacIntosh HG and Hale DE (1976) *Assessment and the Secondary School Teacher.* Routledge and Kegan Paul, London.

3 Bowden R and Jackson N (2002) The principles of assessment. In: Y Carter and N Jackson (eds) *Guide to Education and Training for Primary Care.* Oxford University Press, Oxford.

Index